Designed 2 Eat
The Ultimate Guide To Overall Health for Life

Scott Oteri

"The grading of forms, organic functions, customs and diets showed in an evident way that the normal food of man is vegetable like the anthropoids and apes and that our canine teeth are less developed than theirs and that we are not destined to compete with wild beasts or carnivorous animals."

Charles Darwin

Table of Contents

Introduction

Your Current Level of Health

Proper Balance: The Key to Staying Healthy

Why You Eat Food

Your Lifestyle

How Often Should You Eat?

Drinking Water

Eating The Proper Foods

How Staying Active Helps You Stay Healthy

Eating Outside of the Home

The Benefit of Exercise

Removing the Vices

Major Health Problems in the Western World

Understanding Your Physical Health

Are You At A Healthy Weight?

How Do I Improve My Health?

The Health Care Myth

Food for Healthy Living

Food Is The Biggest Factor!

How Much Do You Need?

How Food Is Processed In The Body

The Stuff Food Is Made Of

Everything You Need To Know About Fat

Reducing Fat in The Diet

How Cholesterol Affects the Body

Facts About Proteins

Everything You Need To Know About Carbohydrates

What You Should Know About Fiber

What You Should Know About Gluten

All About Vitamins

All About Phytochemicals

All About Minerals

The Whole Foods Plant-Based Diet

What to Eat and What To Avoid

Common Questions
The Anatomy of the Human Body
Grains the Wholesome Way
Vegetables for Promoting Health
Fruits The Basis of A Plant-based Diet
Legumes, Nuts, and Seeds
Foods to Increase Your Protein Levels
The Empty Calorie Issue

Everything Your Need To Know About Weight Control
The Importance of Weight Control
How The Whole Foods Plant-based Diet Helps Your Lose Weight
Goal Setting and Weight Loss
How The Body Tells You That You're Full
Adding Regular Exercise

Food As Medicine
Improving Your Health
Reading The Food Labels
Superfoods
Reducing Cardiovascular Disease Risks
Reducing Your Risk For Respiratory Disorders
Eating Right for Digestive Disorders
Reducing Bone and Joint Disorders Through Food
How Your Diet Effects Diabetes
Eating To Reduce the Risk of Cancer

A Whole Food Plant-Based Shopping List
Getting Rid of Your Existing Foods
What to Stock For Breakfast
What to Stock For Lunch
What to Stock for Dinner

Conclusion

Resources

Introduction

There are many different diets that you can participate in, but with so many variations it's often difficult to decipher what's best for overall health. Do you eat gluten, or do you avoid it? Are soy-based products unhealthy, or should your diet revolve around soy? It's easy to get lost in all of the conflicting ideas and decide that you'll focus on health and diet another day.

Fortunately you now own Designed To Eat: The Overall Guide To Health For Life, which sets out to solve the mysteries of great health, one bite at a time. The main purpose of this book is to share with you what scientists, doctors, and health conscious eaters have proven is the healthiest way to eat. All of this information comes from studies and research on the subject that has taken decades to compile.

Figuring out what the right foods to base your diet around shouldn't be a mystery. Unfortunately in today's world food producers and big businesses hide the facts as to what the real basis of a healthy diet is. Now everything is outlined for you so that you have hard facts as to what foods you should eat and what foods to avoid. Soon you'll learn how to decipher a label to determine what nutrients you're really getting from your food.

Get ready to go on a whole new exploration of food. It's sure to change the way you think about what's in your pantry and it'll have you assess whether the foods you have been eating truly are giving you the vital nutrients that your body needs.

Unfortunately the average North American diet consists of too much unhealthy processed foods filled with chemicals and additives.

There's too much reliance on red meats, when there are many great plant-based alternatives out there that provide protein, are low in fat, and reduce the amount of bad cholesterol flowing through the blood.

Simple changes in the average diet can promote positive health, rid the body of disease, and stop the obesity epidemic that has troubled the Western population for years. Diet is the solution to many of the common health problems that are faced in today's modern society.

Too many of the medications that people take on a day-to-day basis are reactive. Not only do those medications not solve underlying problems, but they also create a long list of new ones that often must be solved with medications of their own.

It's time to be proactive to reduce your risk of cancer, cardiovascular disease, and many other problems that plague the Western world. You can solve the problem at the source by demanding the proper nutrients from the food you eat. The foods that you consume should increase your health and well-being, instead of making you overweight and sick.

No diet should rely on foods where nutrients have been stripped away. There shouldn't be overdoses of certain nutrients in your diet while other nutrients are significantly lacking. Solving this matter comes down to knowing the problem exists and educating yourself on the proper way to eat.

I'm here to let you know that you can protect yourself from these problems before they ever begin. This book will teach you everything you need to know about diet and nutrition. Now all you need to do is follow through and experience the benefits for yourself.

Lets begin by taking

inventory of your current level of health.

Your Current Level of Health

The things you do each day influence your level of health. Everything from the combination of foods that you eat and your level of activity determine if you are healthy. Being healthy means that you are comfortable with your body, confident, and not at high risk for disease or health problems. In this section I'll discuss how to promote positive health by eating the right foods, how you can tell whether you are healthy or not, and what you can do to change your health for the best.

Proper Balance: The Key to Staying Healthy

Everything that you put in your body affects your level of health. By eating the right foods, maintaining the proper level of exercise, and understanding your personal food requirements, you ensure that you remain healthy and active throughout life. Ever heard the phrase, "you are what you eat?" That statement is totally correct. By filling your body with nutritious foods you promote health for years to come.

Your body needs a mix of nutrients that include vitamins and minerals, carbohydrates, fats, fiber, and proteins. Getting the proper mix helps your body properly develop, improves your health, and protects you from diseases such as heart disease and cancer. The benefits to eating a well balanced diet are endless. You can reduce your level of stress, improve your mental state, and even positively affect your mood when you eat well. Not eating correctly on the other hand brings about health issues, reduces your amount of energy, and leaves you without the proper nutrients that your body needs.

Food has a direct influence on your weight. So many people in the Western world are obese or overweight, which is a huge risk to the body. Extra weight occurs from eating the wrong foods for the body. If you eat foods that are unhealthy you end up with too much food being stored in your body as fat. If you don't work hard to expend the energy that you receive from your food, you'll pack on the pounds. Balance is key when it comes to eating properly and maintaining your weight. You have to only take in as much as you can exert in order to keep off the pounds.

If you want to lose weight so that you can reduce your risk of diabetes, cancer, cardiovascular disease, and a wide range of other problems, all you have to do is exert more energy than you get from the food you eat. That's the basis of all diet programs. If you have ever failed a diet, you'll learn exactly how to make sure that doesn't happen again and lose the weight for good. In doing so you'll improve your health and maintain it for years to come.

With the correct diet, exercise, and a little willpower, you can learn to avoid the fat and sugary foods that add the extra pounds without providing your body any nutrients. You'll improve your overall level of your physical health, get to a healthy weight, and learn the importance of exercise. Your health all begins with the balance you have when it comes to diet and exercise. It doesn't have to be a difficult process to eat right and be active. Commit to great health and wellness today by starting with the foods you eat.

Why You Eat Food

There are two main reasons that you eat food. The first is to receive all of those crucial nutrients. The second reason you eat is so that your body has enough energy. Your body requires the proper amount of energy to maintain all of its involuntary processes, such as controlling your heart rate and breathing. You also need energy for the voluntary processes, whether that includes you sitting at a desk or running a marathon. Without the proper energy, your body wouldn't be able to function at its highest capacity.

Not getting enough calories through the day results in unhealthy rapid weight loss. This isn't the good form of losing weight since it results in gallstones, created when digestive fluids in your gallbladder harden and bring about severe pain in the body, yellowed skin, and a fever. A calorie deficiency also causes heart problems, loss of concentration, coordination loss, and a ton of other problems. The body is supposed to get the proper energy from the foods you receive.

So since the main purposes of eating food are to give you the correct nutrients and to provide you with enough energy, why would you ever put anything that is unhealthy in it? It makes sense that you would only eat the healthiest foods that add key nutrients to the body and don't include chemical additives, excess sugars and fats, or empty calories.

Next time you eat anything, it's important to ask yourself, "Will this food add or subtract from my level of health?" If the answer is questionable, skip that food source and instead opt for something more nutritious. Do this enough and each time you eat you'll make a conscious decision to promote good energy.

Your Lifestyle

Optimum health can be influenced by your lifestyle. Your lifestyle is a mix of the daily activities you participate in, your eating habits, and any risks that you take with your daily health such as your use of tobacco and alcohol. Lets discuss everything that influences a person's lifestyle.

How Often Should You Eat?

Depending on your lifestyle, you may only be able to eat a couple meals a day, and that's fine. It really depends on the demands of your schedule and your own unique biology. You eat multiple times a day to replenish the amount of energy within the body. Food only gives us enough energy to last for a little while, and then we have to eat and add more nutrients to the body.

The ideal number of main meals you should eat during the day is three. That will give you a steady amount of nutrients so that you have the fuel you need for all of your daily activities. Any less than three times a day and your body will naturally want to choose foods that are high in fat, sugar, and calories. Not eating enough square meals leads to over eating.

You can also add healthy snacks to your diet to help maintain the proper amount of energy. Make sure you stay aware of what's triggering your snacking, whether it's a trigger like seeing food on the TV, thirst, or boredom. Then choose an appropriate snack that is healthy and provides you with enough energy to make it until your next meal. It's possible that you don't even need a snack, and just need to hydrate your body.

Drinking Water

It's pretty common knowledge that your body can only make it for three days without drinking water. Compare that to eating food, which you can live without for several weeks, and you'll understand just how vital water is to the diet.

Your body doesn't have a system for storing water, and it's lost from sweat and urination. Everyday you have to replenish the amount of water in the body so that your body can maintain the proper temperature, support muscles, and help your body get rid of waste.

6 to 8 glasses of water is recommended, but depending on how active your lifestyle is, you may need more. It's good to always have some water on hand and drink a little bit even when you aren't thirsty. Thirst is a signal that your body is already dehydrated from a lack of fluids.

Water is also amazing for dieters. The average American drinks 400 calories a day. That's a pound of fat that you could remove from your body every 9 days by only drinking water instead of sugary drinks. The amount of calories that are in sodas, sweet teas, and fruit juices is one of the biggest causes of weight gain in children, and many of these drinks only add empty calories and extra sugar to the diet.

It can be simple to change your habits when it comes to drinking water. Drink teas and coffee without any added sugar or sweeteners. Carry a bottle of water with you wherever you go, and refill it when you need to. Opt for a drink with less sugar when you're at the store, or just stick to water. Not only will it promote good health, but it will also keep money in your wallet.

Eating The Proper Foods

Do you get the 5 suggested servings of fruits and vegetables a day? For families and individuals it is easy to miss that mark because of fast food, vending machines, and microwave dinners. With the proper diet you'll eat a lot of nutrient rich food that well surpasses the 5 suggested fruit and vegetable serving suggestion.

There are two types of nutrients you receive from the foods you eat. The first type is known as a macronutrient. It includes protein, carbohydrates, and fats. Macronutrients give you energy and are the foundation of a healthy diet. The second type of nutrient is called a micronutrient. These are the vitamins and minerals that you receive from your food. Having the right mix of micronutrients ensures that your body functions properly.

Most foods contain a mix of both macronutrients and micronutrients. When your diet consists of plant-based foods you focus on eating the right blend of foods to have all of your nutrient needs met, which is easily achieved. You'll get the right amounts of carbohydrates, fat, and protein on a plant-based diet. In fact, you'll lower the amount of fat you eat, as well as the amount of sugars, to get only the calories your body requires.

When you begin eating the proper foods you'll notice that you lose or maintain your weight because you're getting just the amount of food and nutrients your body needs. With traditional Western diets you receive too much energy from the foods you consume. All the extra fat and protein you eat ends up adding extra weight. On a plant-based diet you give your body everything it needs, without empty calories or high fat foods.

Eating Outside of the Home

In the Western world, there are many two household families that don't always have time to prepare each meal and instead opt for fast food or pizza parlors. It's suggested that if you are trying to maintain a diet and stay healthy that you either start packing food on the go before hand or opt for healthier foods when you're eating outside of the home.

Most restaurant meals at fast food restaurants have excess fat, are cooked unhealthily, and contain too many calories. If you are going to eat on the go you have to be aware of portion size, levels of sodium and fat, and opt for healthier alternatives. If you really want to promote your health you'll either go to a very healthy restaurant or avoid dining out at all.

How Staying Active Helps You Stay Healthy

There are two primary types of lifestyles, those that are active, and those that are sedentary. A lot of this is influenced by the type of work you do, but it also has to do with how you spend your free time and the activities you participate in.

There are many benefits to maintaining a healthy lifestyle, and you should make decisions that increase your activity level and promote your health. Staying active helps increase your physical well-being and promotes a positive state of mind.

Fitting activity into your life can be as simple as doing extra chores around the house, lawn and garden work, or even walking or biking to work instead of driving. Instead of watching TV when you come home or browsing the internet, why not take a short 30 minute walk? It'll help you lose weight and it's a healthy, cost-free activity.

The Benefit of Exercise

Exercise allows us to maintain our proper health, burns calories, and helps prevent cardiovascular disease and diabetes. It doesn't have to be difficult to get the proper amount of exercise per day and you can achieve your daily exercise goal easily by just changing your normal daily routine a little bit.

A good rule is to aim for 30 minutes of exercise a day. Your exercise doesn't have to be vigorous; you can achieve this goal by briskly walking, swimming, or mowing the lawn. If you are trying to lose weight, it's even better to work out for 300 minutes a week. You can also add in some strength training exercises to build and maintain your strength.

The reason so many people in the western world are overweight has to do with poor eating habits and a lack of exercise. This combination adds on the additional pounds and results in a lot of diseases over time. By eating the correct foods that are low in fat and adding physical exercise, you can lose any excess weight and maintain a healthy lifestyle.

Removing the Vices

The two main vices that affect your health are drinking alcohol and smoking. Reducing or eliminating both of these habits from your life can do wonders for your well-being.

Alcohol doesn't contribute to your nutrition and leads to many different medical conditions. Overconsumption can lead to weight gain, vitamin deficiencies, and depending on your level of consumption even death. It's best to make sure that you control the amount of alcohol you drink. Moderation is best when it comes to drinking.

Smoking is even worse because of the diseases that it is known to cause. Lung cancer, cardiovascular disease, and chronic lung disease are just a few of the possible diseases you're increasing your chances for by smoking or being around secondhand smoke. Once you quit smoking, your overall health is restored within a few months.

Major Health Problems in the Western World

Did you know that more than half of the adult population in America over 20 years of age is overweight or obese? The statistics for children isn't much different. Nearly one-fifth of children and adolescents age 6 -19 are obese. Being overweight or obese can't be blamed on genes. It's a preventable condition that is influenced by food and exercise. Since the population of overweight people continues to increase, that's a sign that the standard diet of a citizen in the United States is failing.

There are two primary reasons that people become overweight. The first reason is due to a diet full of energy-dense food that is high in fat, which results in an individual consuming more calories than they expend. Energy-dense foods are foods that provide a lot of calories with each bite. Some examples of energy-dense foods are processed foods such as your favorite packaged snack food, a cheeseburger at the fast food restaurant your frequent, and meats that are also high in fat.

The second reason people become overweight is from a lack of exercise. At work and school, a lot of time is spent sitting, with very little time moving around and getting the proper exercise. It can also be attributed to economic development, where sitting in a car or on the bus, are often favored to walking or biking to the office. As the economy of a developing country expands, so do its citizens from a mix of less exercise and a higher fat diet. With an overweight population come a lot of related health problems.

Each year hundreds of thousands of people in the United States die of heart disease, cancer, stroke, and diabetes. The greater your body mass, the higher the chance that you will develop one of these diseases. That's why it's vital to improve your level of health, especially if you are overweight. If you think that you are too young to worry about heart failure, cancer, or diabetes, consider the following - each year, thousands of people in each age group die from these diseases. No matter what shape your body is in, you can reverse the negative impact that a poor diet has had on your body.

The secret to feeling younger, living longer, and avoiding disease is all about the food you eat. By changing your diet and the level of physical activity you engage in, you can lose weight and greatly improve your health. When you form good eating habits, you'll lower your risk for many preventable diseases, and you'll physically notice changes in your body too. Overtime you'll feel more alive, you'll lose weight, and you'll notice the common problems you have been taking medication for have disappeared.

So what type of diet will have the highest benefit on your health? It's not a fad, and it's probably not one you hear about too often. It's the Whole Food Plant-Based Diet. Don't let the name fool you. It's a very simple diet to follow, and you get to eat great tasting foods that provide you with all the nutrients you need. Let's discuss the Whole Food Plant-Based Diet in detail.

Understanding Your Physical Health

By learning about your medical health through understanding of your unique lifestyle and your medical history you are able to take charge of your well-being. Uncovering your medical history through both your family genes and based on a medical check up will let you know if you are at risk for any diseases. Once you know any health factors you might face, you can use that information as the basis for improving your health.

You'll want to begin with a medical checkup to learn of any health risks. First your pulse will be taken that will indicate your level of physical fitness. A standard rate for adults is about 60 to 80 beats per minute. You can compare these results with other people in your age category to get a better understanding your overall level of personal health.

Next your blood pressure will be tested. Your blood pressure is a measurement of the pressure of blood in your arteries as your heart pumps. High blood pressure is anything over 140/90mmHg, which can be reduced with proper eating habits, losing weight, and increasing the amount that you exercise.

Depending on your family history, any symptoms you have, and the results of your pulse check and blood pressure, you may also have a blood sample taken. Your blood will be tested for cholesterol levels of both good cholesterol, which is known as high density lipoprotein, and bad cholesterol, called low density lipoprotein. The doctor will also test for triglycerides that exist because of excess calories in the diet, glucose, which informs the doctor whether you have diabetes, and red blood cells in the blood.

All of these tests will explain if you are at high risk for cardiovascular disease and influence if you should follow a diet or increase your amount of exercise.

Are You At A Healthy Weight?

Your distribution of fat and weight in the body explains a lot about the potential problems that can occur in the future. Diet and exercise influence weight distribution, so if you aren't at an ideal weight it's possible to change those with positive eating habits and the proper diet.

People either hold excess weight in their midsection or store fat around their hips and thighs. Having excess weight in the midsection puts you at risk of potential problems. Another way to test you risk is by checking your body mass index results.

Your body mass index (BMI) is a ratio between your height and weight. The higher your BMI number, the more likely you are to be overweight. A BMI of 19 through 24 is considered "normal," but in the Western world it is far from the standard. In America, 2 out of 3 people are overweight and 1 in 3 are obese. Overweight people have a BMI reading of 25 – 30, and obese people have a BMI above 30.

Anyone with a BMI over 25 increases their chances of high cholesterol, high blood sugar, and prehypertension. Having a BMI leads to a higher risk to have a stroke, to develop cardiovascular disease, and to develop diabetes.

If you are overweight or obese then you should make the necessary lifestyle changes to lose weight. Even if you are considering having surgery to shed the pounds, you may be required to lose weight first, so it benefits you to make lifestyle changes immediately.

But How Do I Improve My Health?

Depending on the results of your tests, you may need to change your diet and level of exercise. Plan on not just making these changes temporarily, but instead making them life-long habits.

Even if your tests come out positive, you might still be influenced enough by the teachings in this book to make changes to your diet and exercise regimen. Making the right changes now can ensure your health in the future.

You can choose to make little changes over time or you can make drastic changes all at once. Either way, you have to commit to your changes to see success. If you find yourself slipping up, remember that you can succeed with your diet, and return to it. No one is perfect, but with time you can succeed at increasing your level of health.

Change is a process. As a matter of fact it is a six-step process. It begins before you even think about making a change. It starts one day with you being told that your health isn't as good as it needs to be and forces you to think living healthier. At this point you can decide to make changes to promote your health or you can continue making the same choices you've always made.

Once you have made that decision, your next step is to prepare to follow through with that action. If your goal is to eat healthier, than this step is the planning phase. You prepare by determining what you'll be eating, you write a grocery list, and you plan your meals out for the next week.

After you have successfully prepared to change a habit, next you make the changes you planned to do. In this step you'll purchase the foods on your list and cook the foods that you planned to eat. Once you have done that you are starting to create a habit.

Six weeks after following this process, you've formed a habit. If you break your diet, don't beat yourself up, but instead get right back to it the next day and start to succeed again.

It takes time to focus on improving your health. It's a commitment that you'll have to work hard to achieve. Just know that it is possible to change your lifestyle. Don't hesitate to ask the people around you for support. Change is made one day at a time. Day by day you can influence yourself to make the positive changes that will affect your health.

The Health Care Myth

Even with all of the medical advances that have occurred in the recent years, the death rate in America has stayed around the same level. Everyday you are bombarded with advertisements on television and radio claiming to have the next miracle cure for your ailment. Even though these treatments claim to heal your health condition, many medications have a high risk of side effects that will only bring about a new set of problems.

As a nation the United States spends more money per capita on health care. Even though a lot of money is used for doctor's visits, medications, and trying to achieve peak health, this expenditure isn't trying to prevent people from having the health problem in the first place. Instead the health system is reacting to a problem by trying to cure existing health conditions, which hasn't been working very effectively.

The interesting thing is that scientists and doctors have known for years what the secret is to preventing disease. This secret has been studied numerous times with positive results showing that this one thing not only has the power to reduce your risk of disease, but it can even reverse these conditions. What is that secret? It's not a prescription pill. The secret is how you eat and the diet you maintain.

What type of diet should you maintain? Based on research by Dr. T. Colin Campbell who did a 20 year study on the effects of diet and mortality rates throughout China, where populations of people tended to eat similarly in each county, you should follow the Whole Foods Plant-Based Diet.

The Whole Foods Plant-Based Diet is very simple, and involves only eating foods that are as close to their natural forms as possible. This includes fruits, vegetables, whole grains, beans and legumes, and raw seeds and nuts. With this diet you should avoid all foods that have been processed, animal products, and foods with added salt, sugar, and oil. You want 80% of your calories from carbs, 10% from fats, and 10% from proteins.

So what makes this diet so effective? It's not known for certain, but one theory is when you follow a diet that consists mostly of plant-based foods you counter free radicals that promote cancer and a wide variety of other problems with antioxidants. Antioxidants slow down the aging process in our cells, and promote good health. With animal based products, we lack the proper amount of antioxidants and increase the amount of oxidation occurring in our body which leads to free-radicals that causes cancer and other health conditions.

There you have it. The foods that you eat are more powerful than any prescription drug in the world. Eating the right foods will stop you from having a stroke, migraine headaches, erectile dysfunction and so much more. If you have problems with your weight, if you're taking pills to cure problems and more pills to cure side effects of those first pills, you don't have to live like that anymore. All you need to do is adjust your diet, and you'll feel better than you have in years.

So if your diet is to blame for all of the ailments you're facing, why is it that this information seems to be such a big secret?

The solution is very simple. Healthy eating isn't as profitable for big business. If it's not putting money in the pharmaceutical companies hands, they aren't going to promote it. Instead the truth is hidden behind food and drug companies advertising dollars. Instead of telling you the healthiest way to live, they'd rather promote their unhealthy products to take a piece of your money.

Now you know the secret to good health. Following a Whole Foods Plant-Based Diet can be a gradual change, and doesn't need to be done immediately. Just replacing one meal a day with a Whole Foods Plant-Based Diet alternative can do wonders for your health and is simple to initiate. You'll notice changes in your health and wellness soon after switching from a low nutrient diet and I'll walk you through every step of the way.

Food for Healthy Living

Food Is The Biggest Factor!

The macronutrients are fats, proteins, carbohydrates, and fibers. The amount that you take in on an average day influences the amount of energy you receive from your food. Most food contains a blend of these macronutrients as well as a variety of vitamins and minerals, which are classified as micronutrients.

If you eat foods that provide you with too much energy than you need throughout the day, all the extra calories add weight to your body and overtime you pack on the pounds. If you do this too often then you put yourself at risk for a variety of health problems and diseases. If you eat the right blend of foods, taking into consideration your level of activity, then you'll keep the extra weight down and promote positive health.

With this in mind, you can tell just how important an adequate diet is to your health. Medications don't prevent problems from occurring, but your food will. Healthy eating habits have been proven to increase your overall health, lower your risk of cardiovascular disease, cancer, and many other problems.

If you are wondering why you don't feel as good as you should, or found out that you have a health problem, you should look at your diet and find out how you can improve it. The same can be said if you want to ensure your health and longevity. Start with good eating habits, and over time your body will recover from its current ailments and stop other problems before they ever begin.

How Much Do You Need?

Many different factors determine the amount of calories that you need each day. Your muscle mass plays a large roll in how much energy your body needs. Your gender, age, and even your body temperature are just a few of the factors to take into consideration. Check out this chart to determine a general guideline to how much food you should eat based on your level of activity:

Level of Activity	Calorie Intake
Very Little (Sedentary and Bed Bound)	11.5 calories per pound of body weight
Light	13.5 calories per pound of body weight
Moderate	16 calories per pound of body weight
Vigorous	18 calories per pound of body weight

Now that you know your required level of caloric intake per day, you should also learn how much of each vitamin and mineral is required for optimal health. In North America, you can learn these standards by reviewing the Dietary Reference Intakes (DRI). The DRI suggests how much of each nutrient you should have at a minimum and maximum level based on research. These figures have been published so you know the optimal amounts of vitamins and minerals you should receive in order to prevent disease.

You can learn about the makeup of each food by reviewing its nutrition label. It will explain the calories, vitamins and minerals found in one serving of the food. It will also list all the ingredients used to create the food and display the percentages of protein, carbohydrates, fiber, and fat in each food.

Based on all this information, you can use it as a general guide to understanding how much you need to eat each day, and what amounts of each are considered healthy depending on your specific needs.

How Food Is Processed In The Body

All of the food you eat is broken down chemically so that your body can absorb the nutrients. The whole process begins when you take a bite of food and ends anywhere from a day to three days later once your body releases waste products.

Carbohydrates are either simple sugars or complex carbohydrates that give your body fuel. Simple sugars are just that, foods that are made of a few sugar molecules that are easily digested and quickly enter the bloodstream. This results in a spike in your blood sugar levels that causes your pancreas to produce insulin to remove excess sugar from your body. Once the excess sugar is removed, your body begins to crave more food to increase its blood sugar level again, resulting in a craving for even more sugar. Some examples of foods that become simple sugars are soda, sugar, and maple syrup.

Complex carbohydrates on the other hand take more time to be fully digested but are packed with your body's preferred source of energy. These carbohydrates are converted to glucose that fuels your body, or stored by the body as glycogen, which has the opposite effect of insulin to give you a storage of energy which helps your body function optimally. Complex carbohydrates come from starchy whole grain foods such as brown rice and oatmeal and from fibrous foods like asparagus, spinach, and other leafy vegetables.

Proteins turn into amino acid once broken down, which plays a huge role for your body. Amino acids help you heal from injury, grow, and break down food - among other important processes. Amino acids are the building blocks of biological processes, since they make up a good portion of cells and muscle. Some amino acids known as nonessential amino acids are created in the body, while others called essential amino acids must come from the foods we eat.

When fat is broken down it becomes fatty acid. While most fatty acids provide energy, there is also a type of fatty acid called an essential fatty acid that is required for certain biological processes. These essential fatty acids are omega-3 and omega-6 which comes from fish and vegetable oil respectively.

The Stuff Food Is Made Of

You should already be aware that foods are normally categorized into being a carbohydrate, fat, protein, or fiber. Most foods contain a mixture of these in different proportion. You get amounts of fat, fiber, and protein from whole grain bread, which is considered a carbohydrate. So you don't necessarily have to eat foods that are solely considered as proteins to be getting the proper intake of food.

It's the mixture of everything that you eat and the vitamins, minerals, and nutrients that all of your food provides that contribute to your nutritional intake. No one food group will give you everything you need, which is why a good diet consists of a wide variety of food.

You need a combination of fat, proteins, carbohydrates, fiber, vitamins, and minerals to build a proper diet. What exactly are these things and how can much do you need? All of this is addressed in the upcoming chapters.

Everything You Need To Know About Fat

So what exactly is fat? Fat is a type of lipid that is made from hydrogen, oxygen, and carbon. They exist mostly in meat, plants, and fish. They make up cells that are stored in the body to help with the absorption of nutrients from food, provide energy, and help the body to maintain the proper temperature.

There are different types of fats that play different roles in the body. First you have monounsaturated fats and polyunsaturated fats, which are known as your "healthy fats". Next you have saturated fats and trans fat, which are "unhealthy fats". Too much fat - both healthy and unhealthy - increases the risk of certain diseases in the body.

So what is the difference between the healthy fats and the unhealthy fats? The main differences are the sources of a fat, as well as the chemical make up of both types of fat.

Saturated fat is found in animal and dairy products. Foods like hot dogs, whole milk, and cheese contain high levels of saturated fat.

At room temperature, saturated fats are solid. Excessive intake of saturated fats increases the amount of cholesterol in the blood, which already has enough cholesterol in the body from its production in the liver. In turn this increases your risk of a stroke, heart attack, and coronary heart disease. Foods high in saturated fats are usually also high in calories.

Unsaturated fats on the other hand are found in plant-based foods, and are your healthy fats. Plant foods, fruits and vegetables, and nuts among many other foods are a source of unsaturated fats. At room temperature these fats are liquid. Foods that have unsaturated fat helps the body lower the amount of bad cholesterol in the blood, without lowering the amount of good cholesterol in the body.

There's also a form of fat that you might have heard of called a trans fat. Trans-unsaturated fatty acid is essentially taking an unsaturated fat that is solid and heating it to the point that it's now in liquid form. Once the fat cools it solidifies and becomes your stick or tub of margarine. This type of fat is no different from the saturated fat in the body, and too much of it increases your bad cholesterol. Trans fats are in a lot of different foods that you've eaten. French fries, pies, cake frosting, and so much more kinds of food include some amount of trans fats.

Reducing Fat in The Diet

One important goal to have should be to reduce the amount of fat that you receive in the diet. Not only will it help you cut calories, but it's also healthier for your heart and overall health. You can dramatically cut out the amount of fat in your diet by reducing or eliminating the amount of animal products you eat, changing the methods you

use to cook foods, and by using cooking oil alternatives.

Did you know that beef sausages and hot dogs are 80% fat? On top of it, one-third of that fat is unhealthy saturated fat. The amounts aren't much different for bacon, salami, or chicken hot dogs either. These foods all have a fat percentage over 70%. If you want to reduce the fat in your diet and promote health, you can begin by dramatically reducing the meat you eat, or better yet, by eliminating them altogether.

If you are going to continue eating meat, at a minimum only eat types of meat that have at most a 35% fat to calorie ratio. Saturated fats should not be over 7%, and should ideally be removed from the diet. Sticking to these ratios will reduce your risk for heart disease and keep the pounds off.

Another way to reduce fat from your diet is by changing the way your prepare foods. You don't have to add unnecessary fats to the food you cook by using an alternative method to pan frying or deep-frying. These methods aren't healthy for you and only increase the fat content of your food.

Some alternatives you have are to bake, broil, or pan grill your food. These methods don't require an excessive amount of oil – if any at all. They'll still lock in all of the great flavors, it'll just be the cooking process that has changed, not the result.

If you're going to pan fry, use nonstick pans so that you don't have to add oil to keep your food from sticking. Add wine or lemon juice to foods that require a little more moisture instead of oil. You can also use stock to cook in place of oil.

These subtle changes won't effect how your food tastes, but it will stop you from packing on the pounds. It's changes like this that reduce your risk of heart disease, cancer, and diabetes. On top of it, many of the cooking methods listed above don't take much longer than pan or deep-frying.

How Cholesterol Affects the Body

Cholesterol is a naturally occurring process in the body. It's created in the liver and helps the body produce some hormones, build cell walls, and digest fats. When you have an excess of cholesterol the tissues of your body and organs receive an excess amount of cholesterol.

Plaque can form between the walls of your arteries when you have too much cholesterol in the blood steam making it harder for blood to circulate around your body. If the plaque breaks open it'll form a blood clot. If the blood clot occurs in an artery that sends blood to the brain you'll have a stroke, if it forms in an artery for the heart then the break will cause a heart attack.

For these reasons it's important that your diet does not contain too much saturated fat or too little unsaturated fat. A plant-based food diet reduces the amount of food you're eating which produce bad cholesterol, increase the good cholesterol within the body, which in turn reduces the risk of a blood clot forming in your body and causing a heart attack or stroke.

Since you can combat bad cholesterol by eating the right types of foods and including unsaturated fats in your diet, it's important to know what types of food provides you with necessary unsaturated fat.

There are two types of unsaturated fats. First you have your monounsaturated fats, found in vegetable oils, avocados, nuts and olives. Second is your polyunsaturated fats that you get from fortified foods, which gives you omega-3 fatty acids, and omega-6 fatty acids which comes from vegetable oil, whole-grain foods, and nuts. You should include these types of foods in your diet and replace the foods that provide saturated fats.

Facts About Proteins

Proteins are vital to the body. Your bones, muscle, and skin contain proteins that help it keep its function. Proteins are in every cell in our body and have the ability to repair and maintain each individual cell. There are many different types of proteins that have a wide number of functions. It's a vital part of our chemical makeup and does a lot of good for the body.

When we eat proteins, they are broken down in the body into amino acids. After they are fully digested they enter the bloodstream and provide you with all of the building blocks to produce more proteins in the body.

Overall it is suggested that you eat 46 grams of protein a day if you're a woman, or 56 grams of protein a day if you're a man. This number can be influenced by a number of factors including your amount of exercise, whether you are pregnant, or if you are recovering from malnutrition. If you at a standard health level, those suggested numbers should be an adequate amount of protein for your diet.

Protein doesn't just come from animal products, which are often known for their high protein levels. You also receive protein from whole grain foods, legumes, and other plant-based foods.

It's important to get a wide range of proteins that don't just come from meats. Meats, especially those that are red meat should be limited in the diet in order to reduce the risk of cardiovascular disease. If you are using meat as your primary source of protein then you are missing out on a wide range of healthy foods that provide your body with not only adequate protein amounts, but also include important nutrients that meats don't contain.

It's important to note that it is possible to eat too much protein. Your body isn't able to store protein within the body so when you eat too much it puts an extra workload on the digestive processes that occur in your liver and kidneys. Excess in the proper amount of proteins in the diet can cause kidney disease, a calcium deficiency, and increased saturated fat levels.

The recommended daily amount of protein is 46 – 56g. There's a large misconception that people need tons of protein, which is why it's the basis of most Western diets. The fact is that you can get the correct amounts of protein with a plant-based diet. Your body won't have to store any of the excess animal fat and protein that you're eating, and you'll be at less of a risk for many different diseases and health conditions. Deficiency rarely actually occurs and the only people who are at risk for protein deficiency are either consuming a diet filled with empty calories, or aren't receiving the proper amount of calories with their diet.

Having a protein deficiency signals that you have poor eating habits. Protein deficiency is very uncommon in developed countries and usually only occurs when someone is eating foods that don't supply essential amino acids that the body needs to receive, has a very poor diet, or as someone is recovering from a major trauma.

When most people think about protein rich foods, they normally believe that animal products like meat, dairy, and eggs are the best ways to receive protein. The issue with animal products is the fact they have an excessive amount of fat and lack the important nutrients that a balanced diet requires.

Plant foods on the other hand, do contain all of the proper nutrients in addition to protein that the body needs. You receive dietary fiber and carbohydrates that are missing from animal products when you follow a plant-based diet. By eating the proper types of foods you can get all of the amino acids that your body needs to continue functioning in perfect harmony.

Choose a mix of foods that is healthy and provides you with all of the protein you need. Don't eat an excessive amount of meat and do your best to avoid red meat since it increases the risk for a number of diseases. As long as you follow a diet that is full of the nutrients and vitamins you need, you won't end up being protein deficient or consuming too much protein.

Everything You Need To Know About Carbohydrates

You receive a lot of benefits from the carbohydrates that you eat throughout the day. They give you lasting energy by either becoming simple sugars or complex carbohydrates in the body. These will end up supplying your body with energy and ensure that you brain, tissue, and even cells have what they need. Carbohydrates also help the amino acids in your body produce proteins, build your bones, and create the tissues in your nervous system. It's important to supply your body with the carbohydrates that it needs to do all of these tasks.

You can receive carbohydrates from a variety of foods such as pasta, bread, fruits, vegetables, and legumes. You want to make sure that you choose carbohydrates that come from whole grain products that haven't been refined because most of the nutrients have been removed from refined products, reducing the nutrition level of the food. By eating whole grain foods you'll ensure that you receive enough fiber, protein, vitamins, and minerals that you don't receive with refined products.

Choosing the best carbohydrates means going for healthy alternatives that will provide your body with the correct amount of nutrients. You should receive the carbohydrates in your diet through a variety of fruits, vegetables, and grains to promote your health. Whole grain bread instead of white bread, brown rice instead of white rice, and sweet potato instead of white potatoes are just a few of the improvements you can make to your diet and these choices will in turn improve your health.

What You Should Know About Fiber

There are two types of fiber that create a healthy digestive system and are only found in plant foods. The first type is soluble fiber, which slows the absorption of sugars in the body and helps the stores of energy in your body last longer. The second type is insoluble fiber, which cleans out your system and promotes regular bowel movements.

Soluble fiber turns into gel during the digestion process, attracting water and binding to cholesterol in the body. This interrupts how bad cholesterol is absorbed in your digestive system, and helps to remove excess from the body. With enough soluble fiber in the diet you can reduce your levels of cholesterol and the health effects that come with high levels of bad cholesterol.

Soluble fiber also slows the digestive process, making you feel like you are full longer and helping you to maintain a healthy weight. Since it also slows sugar absorption, soluble fiber reduces the blood sugar levels in the body, which can help control diabetes. You can receive soluble fiber from fruits, vegetables, and grains like oats.

Insoluble fiber works like a laxative to help food and waste pass through your system. Unlike with soluble fiber, insoluble fiber isn't digested, and instead travels through the gastrointestinal tract whole, speeding up the process of having a bowel movement and keeping your system cleaned out. Water is attracted to the insoluble fiber, which causes your stool to be softer and easier to pass.

You should be taking in anywhere from 25 to 40 grams of fiber each day, but most people in the Western world eat much less than that. It comes down to making poor choices about the foods they eat and not introducing enough fiber rich plant-based foods into the diet.

The benefits of a fiber rich diet is that with enough of these foods you'll feel full sooner and longer, which helps with anyone tying to manage their weight. It slows the release of insulin into the blood and the food you eat provides you with energy throughout the day instead of for just a little while then causing you to crash.

It also helps clean out your system and fights constipation by promoting regular bowel movements. This can help reduce your chance of colorectal cancer, increase the amount of gut flora in the body that helps the colon, and stops you from developing any diverticular disease.

If you aren't getting enough fiber, increase your intake overtime. Eat enough fruits and vegetables, add whole grain products to your diet, and add oats to your food.

Balance out the increased levels of fiber with enough water to promote a healthy digestive system.

What You Should Know About Gluten

There's been a lot of concern about whether you should consume gluten or not. Gluten is a form of protein that is found in wheat, rye, and barley. Some people such as those who suffer from Celiac disease should absolutely not consume gluten. Others who are sensitive to gluten should cut back on the amount of whole wheat that they consume in your diet. Most people however don't have gluten intolerance and whole wheat should be a decent portion of what you eat with the whole foods plant-based diet.

When people with Celiac disease consume small amounts of gluten, it triggers an immune response that stops other nutrients from being absorbed in food and damages the small intestine.

When there is a reduction in the amount of nutrients being absorbed by the body, this causes a lot of significant health problems. Those who are sensitive to gluten face the same problems from consuming foods with gluten in it but without the intestinal damage.

Most people don't receive enough fiber in your diet, and when you cut out whole grain foods, you reduce the amount of fiber you get even further. Unless you are sensitive to gluten or have Celiac disease, you don't need to cut back on gluten. A gluten free diet isn't going to be what helps you lose weight. If you're not sensitive to gluten, the most important thing you can do is maintain a healthy diet with a variety of whole foods that are plant based to get enough of the nutrients you need.

All About Vitamins

Vitamins are chemical substances that are in foods, created within the body, and obtained through sunlight. Vitamins are essential to life since they promote growth and development of the body. It aids in the processing of the foods that we eat, builds cells and tissues, and causes chemical reactions within the body.

There are two types of vitamin deficiencies, primary and secondary. If you don't receive enough vitamins from the food that you eat then you have a primary deficiency. A secondary vitamin deficiency is caused by your lifestyle habits such as excessive alcohol consumption, disease, or using medications that reduce the effectiveness of the body in processing vitamins. In the Western world it is unlikely that vitamin deficiencies exist.

Overdosing on vitamins from food sources is very rare, but it often happens as a result of taking too many vitamin supplements. Check with your doctor before increasing your standard dose of any vitamins, otherwise you could end up facing some health issues as a result of an overdose.

The best way to receive your vitamins is by increasing the variety of foods you eat. Most people limit what they eat and purchase at the supermarket to only a few foods. Changing the foods you normally eat can make sure that you get a wide range of vitamins in the diet.

Fresh foods have the highest amounts of vitamins immediately after they have ripened and are picked Frozen is a good alternative since frozen foods are picked at their ripest and flash frozen with all of the nutrients locked in. Cook your foods as minimally as possible to ensure that you are getting as much of the nutrients as you can from your foods.

Lets break down all of the vitamins, the amounts of vitamins that you should get daily, and what happens when you are deficient of that vitamin:

Vitamin A
Daily Requirements: Men 900RAE, Women 700RAE

Vitamin A is one of three antioxidants, which also includes vitamins C and E. Antioxidants reduce the risk of certain cancers. Vitamin A is crucial for sight, healthy bone growth, healthy skin and mucous membranes, and for reproduction.

Vitamin A is received from animal products and plant products in two different varieties. Active forms of vitamin A, known as retinoids are from animals, and provitamins are from fruits and vegetables that are yellow, orange, and dark green, which are known as carotenoids. Provitamins have to be converted in the body into an active form of vitamin A.

Your body stores vitamin A for later use. The liver holds and releases vitamin A, and it is carried to cells and tissues within your body via your bloodstream. If you lack the proper vitamin A in the body, you'll suffer from eye disorders that could cause night blindness or irreversible blindness. Growth problems, the inability for your skin to heal properly, and skin rashes are common in people who lack the proper amount of vitamin A.

You can receive enough vitamin A by eating sweet potatoes, carrots, collard greens, and other dark green, yellow, and orange fruits and vegetables.

Vitamin B6
Daily Requirements: 1.3mg for both men and women

Vitamin B6 assists in the production of amino acids from protein. It helps your body produce insulin, antibodies, and chemicals. Vitamin B6 also relieves symptoms of a number of disorders, and can help reduce the risk of cardiovascular disease.

Deficiency occurs when levels of vitamin B6 are reduced in the body from medications, alcohol abuse, smoking, and oral contraceptives for women. It can cause depression, oily skin, confusion, and a number of other problems.

You can get enough vitamin B6 in your diet by eating potatoes, sweet potatoes and bananas.

Vitamin B12
Daily Requirements: .0024mg for both men and women

Vitamin B12 promotes healthy growth in children, helps create healthy red blood cells, processes carbohydrates and fats, and is needed by the nervous system in creating DNA and genes. It enters your blood stream through binding with a protein known as intrinsic factor in the stomach.

You can receive vitamin B12 through fortified foods such as breakfast cereal, from nutritional yeast, and from other food products. It's available in most multivitamins, and in plant based sources like spirulina, barley grass, and seaweed as well.

A deficiency of vitamin B12 can cause anemia, nerve damage, and dementia. People whose bodies cannot produce intrinsic factor, those whose bodies have stopped creating gastric acid and pepsin, and those with an excess of stomach bacteria should take a supplement.

Vitamin C
Daily Requirements: Men 90mg, Women 75mg

Vitamin C is not manufactured in the body and must be received by eating certain foods. It's easily removed from food through food processing and cooking because of how unstable it is. Vitamin C is important in strengthening bones, repairing the tissues and wounds of the body, and for body growth. It is an antioxidant that allows white blood cells fight against infection, produces red blood cells, and helps the body with iron absorption.

If you don't eat the proper foods, you will end up with a vitamin C deficiency. Vitamin C levels are reduced in the bodies of regular drinkers and smokers. Without enough vitamin C you may end up with scurvy that causes a lot of other issues to the body.

You can find vitamin C in asparagus, plantain, broccoli, oranges, and many other fruits and vegetables. Choose sources that you can cook minimally or don't require cooking at all so that the vitamin C isn't removed from your foods.

Vitamin D
Daily Requirements: 0.005mg for men and women

There are two forms of vitamin D, known as vitamin D2 and vitamin D3. D2 is found in a few different foods, while D3 is created from exposure to the sun. Both D2 and D3 are converted to an active form so that it can be used in your body's kidneys and liver.

The body with the help of vitamin D uses and absorbs calcium and phosphorus. If calcium levels are reduced in your body then vitamin D will convert to its active form and stimulate the body to absorb more calcium and phosphorus. This process ensures that your bones, teeth, and cartilage remain healthy.

You can receive vitamin D by exposing yourself to sunshine. If you don't get enough vitamin D you risk having vitamin D deficiency. Vitamin D deficiency causes softening of the bones and results in bones breaking easily, pain throughout the body, and deformity of the bones in children.

Vitamin E
Daily Requirements: 0.015mg for men and women

Vitamin E, along with vitamins A and C are antioxidants and help rid the body of free radicals. Free radicals oxidize the proteins, fats, and DNA in the body cells and tissues. Vitamin E stops too many free radicals from building up in the body, prevents blood clots, and helps make red blood cells.

Vitamin E is stored within the body, mostly in the liver. If you don't have enough then your nervous system can stop functioning as well, and anemia can be caused. It's pretty rare to have a deficiency of vitamin E.

You can get vitamin E by eating nuts, shrimp, wheat germ, and soybeans.

Vitamin K
Daily Requirements: Men 0.12mg, Women 0.09mg

Vitamin K reduces the ability of blood to clot. It's stored in the liver, and produced within the body by gut flora that lives in the intestine. It can also be found in fruits and vegetables like asparagus, broccoli, grapes, and pears.

A deficiency can occur for a number of reasons, including antibiotic use and any condition that changes how well our bodies absorb fats. If you are deficient in vitamin K, you'll notice that you're bleeding from various parts of your body, that your skin bruises easily, and there's an increase risk of blood clots.

Biotin
Daily Requirements: 0.03mg for men and women

Biotin is a B-complex vitamin that is crucial for turning our food into forms that the body can use. It's commonly used to help with the symptoms of depression, hair loss, and diabetes.

If you don't have enough biotin in your body then you may face hair loss, mental problems, loss of appetite, and other serious symptoms. Biotin can be found in peanuts, black-eyed peas, yeast, mushrooms and cauliflower.

Folic Acid
Daily Requirements: 0.4mg for men and women

Folic acid plays a roll in building DNA, RNA, in new cell production and in healthy growth and development. It is not created within the body, requiring you to consume foods as a source of folic acid, or to take a supplement.

Deficiency of folic acid is a result of a poor diet, a side effect from certain medications, and a result of aging. A folic acid deficiency is common with people who eat processed foods and foods that are high in fat, without eating the right amount of fruits and vegetables.

Without enough folic acid in your system your system is at risk of megaloblastic anemia, weight loss, heartburn, and cardiovascular disease among other issues. You can find folic acid in green vegetables, oranges, beans, and many other fresh foods.

Niacin
Daily Requirements: Men 16mg, Women 14mg

Niacin creates many different chemical reactions within the body to produce energy. It also helps produce and breakdown fats and amino acids, develop and maintain the nervous system, and manufacture DNA. It has been used to treat high blood-cholesterol levels in low doses.

You can find niacin in protein rich foods such as kidney beans, peanuts, soybeans, green peas, meats, poultry, and fish. You're at risk of having niacin deficiency if you drink excessive amounts of alcohol, which can reduce the ability of your body to absorb niacin and if you are deficient in vitamin B6 since B6 is used to convert niacin in the body.

Pellagra is a vitamin deficiency disease that is caused by low levels of niacin. It causes weakness, anxiety, and irritability at its earlier stages. If it is allowed to develop the symptoms then cause skin rashes, diarrhea, delirium, and even death.

Pantothenic Acid
Daily Requirements: 5mg for men and women

Pantothenic acid is also known as vitamin B5. It assists in the breaking down of proteins, creation of vitamin B12, and manufacturing of cell membranes. This vitamin is made in the body, and can also be received from sweet potatoes, red meats, fish, beans, lentils, avocado, and mushrooms. There isn't normally deficiency in the body of pantothenic acid.

Riboflavin
Daily Requirements: Men 1.3mg, Women 1.1mg

Riboflavin is also known as vitamin B2. It helps turn

carbohydrates into energy, digest fats, protects the nervous system and assists the body. You can get enough riboflavin by eating asparagus, okra, meat, and dairy products.

Being deficient in riboflavin can create issues of the mouth and throat, bloodshot and itchy eyes, and mouth ulcers. You are usually deficient of riboflavin because you don't have the appropriate diet or because your body cannot absorb this vitamin in the intestine.

Thiamine

Daily Requirements: Men 1.2mg, Women 1.1mg

Thiamine is known as vitamin B1 and helps create the energy your body needs from carbohydrates and fats. Enough B1 in your body helps regulate your heart, nervous, and digestive systems. You can receive enough thiamine by eating green peas, spinach, navy beans, nuts, pinto beans, soybeans, and red meats.

A thiamine deficiency causes weight loss, poor appetite, and fatigue at its early stages. If the thiamine deficiency continues then it can cause nerve damage, rapid heart rate, and headaches.

Beriberi is also a form of thiamine deficiency that affects people who have a high intake of alcohol, babies who are breast-fed and have thiamine deficiency, and people whose dies primarily consists of carbohydrates that are lacking in thiamine. Beriberi causes nervous system problems and heart failure.

All About Phytochemicals

If you want to protect your body, one way to do that is by eating enough plant-based foods. Plant-based foods have phytochemicals, which are naturally protective chemicals. You can find it in whole grain foods, vegetables like broccoli, Brussel sprouts, and cauliflower, citrus fruits, and even wine.

There are as many as 100 phytochemicals in a single serving of vegetables. The health benefits of having diets filled with phytochemical rich foods are immense. Below is a list of a few of the different phytochemicals and what you can eat to receive their benefits:

Bioflavonoids – Helps you absorb vitamin C. Found in citrus fruits.

Carotenoids – Protects against cardiovascular disease. Found in sweet potatoes, butternut squash, and carrots.

Flavonoids – Protects the body from infection and found in a wide range of foods.

Glucosinolates – Helps detoxify the body, reduces tumor growth, and helps make the body immune. Found in vegetables.

Indoles – Helps with breast cancer and cancer prevention. Found in cruciferous vegetables.

Isoflavones – Fights against estrogen-promoted cancer and lowers cholesterol levels. Found in legumes.

Limonoids – Protects lung tissue, inhibits forms of cancer. Found in citrus fruits.

Lycopene – Protects against types of cancers and against cardiovascular disease. Found in tomatoes.

Organosulfides – Boosts the immune system, stimulates cancer enzymes, delays blood clot formation. Found in onions.

Para-coumaric acid – Helps prevent cancer. Found in tomatoes, carrots, peanuts and other plant-based foods.

Phenols and polyphenol – Protects from chemical damage. Found in many fruits and grains.

Phytoestrogens – Protects against cardiovascular disease. Found in soy and flaxseed.

Phytosterols – Lowers cholesterol levels. Found in soy-based products.

Terpenes – Blocks cancer-causing carcinogens. Found in many plant foods.

All About Minerals

Minerals are substances that are in rocks and metal ores, passed to you through the minerals in the soil. Minerals are necessary for your health and come in two main categories depending on the quantities your body needs.

Minerals that make up more than .005 of your body weight are known as macrominerals and you require more than 100mg of this in our diet daily. The macrominerals are calcium, chloride, magnesium, phosphorus, potassium, sodium and sulfur.

Microminerals make up less than .005 of your body weight and you require less than 100mg daily. Microminerals are also known as trace elements and include chromium, copper, fluoride, iodine, iron, selenium, and zinc.

Minerals play a number of roles in the body such as regulating metabolism, creating chemical reactions to break down foods, and for cell functioning. Your body stores minerals that it can use later in case of a dietary deficiency. If you aren't getting enough calcium, iron, or iodine in your diet, your body may keep enough of these minerals to use years later.

The best sources of minerals are animal products, fruits, and vegetables. Organic foods and foods that have not been processed are the best sources of nutrients, since many different minerals are lost in the refinement process, and because of pesticides.

Since minerals can easily be lost in the refinement process, US law requires that certain minerals be replaced in the food. This is why there are many different enriched foods. Unfortunately not all of the nutrients that are lost will be replaced in enriched foods.

Minerals are removed during the cooking process, especially when we boil nutrient rich foods. For this reason you should try and keep the cooking time down for nutrient rich foods, or find an alternative method to boiling, such as steaming. You can also reuse the water that you boil the food in for soup stock.

If you don't receive the proper amount of nutrients because of the foods you eat (or don't eat,) then you should take a daily supplement to ensure your body gets everything it needs. You'll prevent future health issues and make sure that the mineral reserves aren't depleted in your body, and that the minerals are saved for a time when your body needs them.

Lets breakdown the different minerals and what happens if your body doesn't receive enough of each one:

The Macronutrients

Calcium
Daily Requirement: 1000mg for men and women

Calcium is present in bones and teeth, which make up a majority of the calcium found in the body. The rest is used in blood clotting to protect you from bleeding to death if you have a wound, for nerve signaling, and to contract muscles.

A deficiency of calcium takes years to discover since the body continues to tap into the reserves from your bones. Deficiency causes osteoporosis, bone pains, and muscle cramps.

You can receive calcium from green leafy vegetables, almonds, and tofu.

Chloride
Daily Requirement: 2000mg for men and women

Chloride helps to keep your body fluids level and helps create hydrochloric acid which are digestive juices that line your stomach.

Although it is rare, chloride deficiency can occur when you lose too much liquid from your body. A deficiency results in your body becoming too alkaline, which leads to a number of health issues.

It's very simple to ensure you receive enough chloride since it is a main part of table salt. You can also find it in vegetables like celery and seaweed.

Magnesium

Daily Requirement: 420mg for men, 320mg for women

Magnesium creates nerve signals to control muscle contractions, assists the body in processing fats and proteins, and plays a role in regulating the amount of calcium in the blood. It's stored in your bones and muscles.

Deficiency is a rare but can come about from alcohol abuse, as a result of diseases of the liver, or when the intestine has difficulty absorbing magnesium for the body. When you are deficient in magnesium it causes your blood to also have low calcium and potassium, and causes changes in the heart and nervous system. The problems that a magnesium deficiency causes can be fatal so it's best to treat it when you notice your body having impaired speech, tremors, or irregular heart rhythms.

You can receive enough magnesium including whole grains, nuts, legumes, green leafy vegetables, and tofu in your diet.

Phosphorus

Daily Requirement: 700mg for men, 700mg for women

Phosphorus is needed for a number of important processes throughout the body. It plays a role in healthy teeth and bones, helps the body store energy, and is found in your DNA. The more phosphorus you need, the more that your body will absorb this mineral through the foods you eat.

Having a phosphorus deficiency isn't uncommon for people who take a lot of antacids. If you notice muscle weakness, kidney stones, or bone pain, a lack of phosphorus may be the cause.

Introduce whole grains, legumes, nuts, and sunflower seeds to your diet to reduce your risk of a phosphorus deficiency. Getting enough vitamin D also helps your body to absorb phosphorus.

Potassium

Daily Requirement: 3500mg for men and women

Potassium helps maintain the correct level of fluids in the body, and makes sure that the PH levels aren't to acidic or alkaline. It helps to give your muscles, heart, kidneys, and adrenal valves the proper amount of energy to function.

Potassium leaves the body through sweat, yet potassium deficiency is still uncommon. You are at risk of potassium deficiency if you have kidney disease, an eating disorder, or take too many laxatives that stop the body from absorbing the proper amounts of potassium.

Potassium deficiency is called hypokalemia this disease can cause problems in your heart and kidney. You'll also notice cramps, constipation, and muscle weakness.

Whole grains, potatoes, bananas, cantaloupe, oranges, and lima beans are among many foods that have high levels of potassium. Including these foods in your diet can reduce your risk of stroke, osteoporosis, and kidney stones.

Sodium

Daily Requirement: 500mg for men and women

Like potassium, sodium also regulates body fluid levels and the acidity of blood. It also with transmitting nerve signals and muscle contractions.

Since sodium is in most foods, especially processed foods, getting enough of this mineral usually isn't an issue. In fact it's more likely that you receive too much sodium through your diet. Overtime this overdose results in high blood pressure, heart failure, and other problems.

If you become deficient on the other hand due to illness or dietary problems, you may begin to get cramps, headaches, fatigue, and even fall into a coma.

Sulfur

Daily Requirement: 800 – 1000mg for men and women

Sulfur helps turn proteins into amino acids and carbohydrates into energy. It also helps build healthy skin and produces different vitamins in the body. Sulfur is present in all foods naturally, so there's no risk of not getting enough of it in your diet.

Leafy green vegetables, legumes, and nuts all contain large amounts of sulfur.

The Micronutrients

Chromium

Daily Requirement: 0.035mg for men, 0.025mg for women

Chromium works with insulin to promote healthy levels of blood sugars throughout the body. It also has an influence on the metabolism of fats, carbohydrates, and proteins.

Deficiency can occur as a result of physical stress, pregnancy, and for people with diets high in simple sugars. Most likely it will occur if you are being fed intravenously, which might cause diabetes like symptoms if chromium is not introduced to the food you're eating.

You can get chromium from broccoli, potatoes, green beans, and fruits.

Copper

Daily Requirement: 0.9mg for men and women

Copper plays a wide role throughout many different processes. It helps with positive growth, is an antioxidant, and helps form red blood cells. Copper deficiency is rare, but leads to anemia.

You can receive enough copper by eating whole grains and nuts.

Fluoride

Daily Requirement: 4mg for men, 3mg for women

Fluoride helps maintain healthy teeth by reducing the chances of having tooth decay. You can get it through drinking water or by eating food that is prepared in water that has been fluoridated. Lack of fluoride can lead the higher risks of tooth decay, which you can reduce by using toothpaste or mouthwash with fluoride in it.

Iodine

Daily Requirement: 0.15mg for men and women

Much of your body has iodine in it. A little less than half of the iodine in your body is stored in the thyroid gland where thyroid hormones are produced. These hormones are used by the body to promote growth and metabolism.

Deficiency of iodine stops the proper hormones in the thyroid gland from being created. If this happens the thyroid gland will enlarge, and cause goiter or cretinism. Goiter is when your neck swells because of a enlarged thyroid gland. Cretinism causes dwarfism and mental difficulties due to reduced growth and development in children.

Iodine is found naturally in the sea and we find iodine in our diet from salt that has been fortified with iodine and from plants that were grown near the ocean.

Iron

Daily Requirement: 8mg for men, 18mg for women

Iron is only needed in small quantities, yet it plays an important role of helping transport oxygen throughout the body. It also helps to release energy to the body through the intestines.

Iron deficiency is a common problem that can easily be fixed. Iron in animal products is easier for humans to absorb than iron from plant products. Vitamin C however will remedy this and allow the body to absorb more iron from plant-based foods.

You can include iron in your diet by eating spinach, legumes, and dried fruit.

Selenium

Daily Requirement: 0.055mg for men and women

Selenium is another mineral that acts as a antioxidant to protect your body from free radicals. It helps maintain the immune system and thyroid gland.

Selenium deficiency is rare since the daily requirements are so low. You can include selenium into your diet by eating whole wheat, brown rice, and Brazil nuts. There's also a chance the selenium can help reduce the risk of cancer.

Zinc

Daily Requirement: 11mg for men, 8mg for women

Zinc plays a role in forming DNA, RNA, and the cells in your body. It also helps the body to develop, reproduce, and heal.

Not having enough zinc in your diet can cause health problems including growth problems with children, hair loss, delayed sexual maturation, and digestive problems among other things.

You can receive the proper amount of zinc in your diet by eating navy beans, soy beans, and oat bran.

Now that you understand everything you need to know about vitamins, minerals, and phytochemicals, lets discuss a specific diet that ensures you eat the foods that are healthy for your body.

The beauty of this diet is that you can eat foods without the need to focus on receiving a certain nutrient from the food you eat. All you have to do is get the proper amount of calories and you'll be able to rest assured that your body has gained all the nutrients it needs.

As you can tell, everything that you put in your body has a direct impact on your health. With the diet outlined in the next section, you'll supply your body with the right foods to fight disease, reverse the effects of bad eating habits, and lose or maintain your weight. Let's get into it!

The Whole Foods Plant-based Diet

A whole food plant-based diet can help reduce your risk of disease, help you lose weight, and improve your health. It is the natural way of eating that has promoted health in humans for centuries. Until now there hasn't been any talk about the type of foods you can eat on this diet, so I want to relieve your stress about wondering if a whole food plant-based diet can work for you.

You should have an understanding of why you eat and what foods you should avoid eating. Next you'll learn exactly what you can and cannot have while following a whole food plant-based diet. The great thing about the whole foods plant-based diet is that you can eat the foods that you love to eat. How you prepare and cook them will be different, but you meals will still be satisfying and delicious.

Essentially whole foods are foods that have not undergone any significant changes or processing. Instead of getting chemicals and additives, you're receiving nutritious food the way it's supposed to be eaten, fresh and unaltered. There won't be any added artificial ingredients to your food and it will be all-natural. You can still add a little salt and sugar to food, you'll just receive healthier level of those substances. Eating whole foods ensures that you receive all of the food's nutrients without losing it through processing.

Have you ever taken a look at the ingredient list of the foods that are in your refrigerator and pantry? Chances are that if most of the food you eat even has a label in the first place, that it has undergone some form of processing. If there are a lot of ingredients that you can't pronounce or you're unsure what they even are, then that food item has gone through a lot of food processing.

So why do processed foods exist? Throughout time humans have tried to extend the shelf life of food. Since foods are seasonal, and many go bad very quickly, processing food is a way to store the food for a longer amount of time. Ingredients are added so that the food keeps longer on the shelf and to add convenience. Processed foods are fast and inexpensive to prepare, which works well for a hustle and bustle lifestyle. Processed foods also manipulate the taste of the food by adding flavoring and extra salt.

Even though these are logical reasons to process food, there are also downsides to the processing of foods. When food is altered, it loses in high levels of nutritional value. The vitamins, minerals, and fiber that you get from processed food are only a small portion of what you would receive from a whole food alternative.

Even food that has been fortified or enriched to add new nutrients or to replace nutrients that were lost in the manufacturing process cannot compare to whole foods. A white bread may add certain nutrients, but still doesn't compete health-wise against whole grain bread. Processing just removes too much of the great nutrients that our bodies require.

In addition to removing nutrients while processing foods, unhealthy ingredients are also included to the mix. Cost is a huge factor for food companies, and they are always trying to reduce the expense of creating foods by using unhealthy ingredients. High fructose syrup and soy oil are one such example. These types of foods are subsidized by the government, add no nutrients to the food whatsoever, and add nothing but fat and sugar to our diet.

The basis of most diets is filled with unhealthy foods and significantly lacking in foods that are vitamin and nutrient rich. There's too much dependence on foods that are high in fat, energy, and salt, and not enough fruit, vegetables, and whole grains in the diet. There's even proof that overtime the levels of nutrients in your food is being reduced because of soil depletion, meaning that you have to focus on making sure you get all of the proper vitamins and minerals from your food.

By cutting out the processed foods from your diet, you start receiving vital nutrients and reduce the unhealthy additives. You're left with food the way that it's supposed to be – natural and fresh.

What to Eat and What To Avoid

So what can you eat on a whole foods plant-based diet? Here's a list of the foods that you'll be eating regularly:

Fruits
Vegetables
Whole Grains
Tubers and Starchy Vegetables
Legumes

With a whole food plant-based diet you are eating unrefined or minimally refined plants. Your food won't contain any dyes, artificial ingredients, chemical preservatives or artificial ingredients.

The foods you will exclude:

Meat
Dairy Products
Eggs
Refined Food like oil, bleached flour, and refined sugar

Essentially with a whole food plant-based diet you are reducing or removing the foods that cause health problems such as your red meat, your dairy products, and your refined foods, and replacing it with the food that naturally heals the body, you fruits, vegetables, and whole grains.

You really have a lot of freedom with this type of diet. You don't need to plan out the meals you eat trying to get benefits from single nutrients that are found in a specific food. Instead you eat a variety of plant-based whole foods that will easily get you all of the nutrients you need in better proportions than when you eat a animal-based or processed foods diet.

You also don't limit yourself to just green leafy foods. Yes, you eat vegetables in your diet, but that's not the basis of your diet. It's just a portion of it. The rest of your diet is filled with foods starchy foods, whole grains, fruits, and beans. You're able to prepare your favorite foods and eat what you like.

You can still make comfort foods you enjoy. The way you prepare them might change, but you're able to cook great tasting food that you'll enjoy eating.

Common Questions

Now that I have introduced the main focus with this diet, I think that I should answer some of the common questions that people have. Hopefully this will clear up any of the concerns you have about beginning this diet.

Will I Get Enough Protein on this Diet?
The most common question is about the protein levels your body will receive on a whole foods plant-based diet. Most people believe that you can only get enough protein through consumption of meats and animal products. That's simply a myth that should be dispelled. Meats and animal products do contain large amounts of protein. The issue is that there's too much protein in animal products and as a result the

average American receives three to five times more protein then required to maintain optimal health.

As long as you are eating the correct amount of calories that your body needs, it's nearly impossible to be protein deficient. If you are getting enough calories but are calorie deficient, it means that there is a problem with your diet. You are either eating nothing but foods that are low in protein such as a diet of only apples, a diet of nothing but sugars and fats, or only alcohol.

With a plant-based whole foods diet, you'll eat a variety of foods, get the calories you need, and easily eat the correct amount of proteins. In fact you'll receive much healthier levels of protein then you would with an animal product diet. This will promote good health and reduce the risk of diseases that come with an overload of fat and protein in the body.

Don't I Need Animal Products Like Dairy to Get Enough Calcium? Another myth people have is that dairy is the only way to get the proper level of calcium. Yes, dairy products have a lot of calcium and can provide you with the daily value of calcium you need in small quantities. The problem is that the acidity of dairy products actually causes your bones to use more calcium than it gains and causes bone disease.

Most people don't realize that consuming dairy products isn't the only way to receive calcium. It's abundant in a wide range of foods, many of which you'll be eating with a whole foods plant-based diet. Animal proteins and dairy has been shown to increase the risk of cancer and autoimmune disease. It also plays a roll in heart disease and stroke, so it's best if you avoid dairy and animal products altogether.

Calcium is your body's most abundant mineral. It's also common in animal products because animals eat plants that are rich in calcium, and it's metabolized into their bodies and passed on to us. Instead of consuming calcium from animals, we'll return directly to the source and eat plenty of whole foods that have an abundance of calcium and contribute to healthy bones.

There are two ways that calcium is removed from the body, which entirely depends on your diet. The first way is by consuming an acidic diet, and the second is by receiving too much sodium from your food. With a whole foods plant-based diet, you won't rely on foods that are only acidic or only alkalizing, but instead get full variety of foods that provide you with the proper balance. You'll also lower your sodium intake by not relying on processed foods that are high in salt to provide you with all of your daily nutrients.

Why Am I Avoiding Oil? Olive oils and other types of vegetable oils are constantly being called "heart healthy" and said to promote overall health. Unfortunately, this just isn't the case. Yes, replacing butter with vegetable oils will reduce your amount of bad cholesterol in the body however it won't provide you that much of a health benefit.

Oil is nothing but fat and a ton of calories. All of the nutrients from the vegetable before production have been wasted, and your body cannot tell that it is receiving any calories from oils, even though they have more calories per gram than any other food. Consuming oils leads to over-eating and has a negative impact on the heart by promoting heart disease and increasing the risk of cancer.

Should I Take Fish Oil Supplements?

On a whole foods plant-based diet you don't need to

take fish oil supplements for the omega-3 fatty acids. You can actually get enough of your omega-3 fatty acids from plant-based foods like green leafy vegetables, walnuts, soybeans and ground flaxseed meal.

Too much animal oils are never good. Even though fish oils are known as good oil, it can still raise your cholesterol; increase free radicals in the body, and negatively influence the immune system.

Fish don't produce omega-3 fatty acids themselves; it's actually a byproduct of the food that they eat. If you are worried about not getting enough omega-3 fatty acid in your diet, consider purchasing a supplement that comes directly from the algae and plankton that supplies the fish with their omega-3.

What Nutrients Will My Diet Lack?

The only nutrient you should make sure you get enough of is vitamin B12, which is not found reliably in plant foods. Vitamin B12 helps the nervous system and without it, there's a risk of blindness, deafness, and dementia. It is created by bacteria when manure fertilized soil is digested and broken down within animals.

Over the years, excess vitamin B12 is stored in your body, and can last for years. That isn't to say that you should stop getting enough vitamin B12. Most animal products don't give you enough vitamin B12, but there are a couple options you have to add it to your diet.

So how do you receive enough vitamin B12? Make sure that you eat foods that have been fortified with vitamin B12. You can also drink milk alternatives such as almond milk and soymilk that has been fortified with vitamin B12. Nutritional yeast, vegan mayonnaise, and many types of cereals have been fortified with B12 as well.

Do I Need To Eat Organic Products?

It's up to you as to whether you'd like to purchase organic products or not. Many of these foods are more expensive, and cost should not stop you from following a whole foods plant-based diet. The main concern of the diet is getting enough healthy food, and reducing the amount of foods that have been proven to cause disease, not whether it's organic or not.

The Anatomy of the Human Body

Human beings haven't always consumed meat and animal products, and our physiology proves it. Here are some of the common differences between your makeup and the makeup of carnivores:

Teeth

Carnivores and omnivores have long pointed teeth for ripping into meat and tearing raw flesh. Herbivores have flat teeth so that they can grind their food, instead of eating it whole.

Jaws

The jaws of carnivores and omnivores only move up and down, not side to side like herbivores do. This allows herbivores to chew their food instead of eating it whole, just like their teeth do.

Saliva

The salivary glands of carnivores and omnivores are small and don't help brake down food with digestive enzymes. They can't predigest their own foods. Herbivores on the other hand have complex salivary glands that produce alkaline saliva to digest food even before it reaches the stomach.

Intestines

A small intestine of a carnivore and omnivore is small so that waist can travel through the intestines quickly to reduce the amount of rotting waste in the digestive system. Herbivores have small intestines that are longer and winds back and forth throughout the body to allow all of the nutrients to absorb into the system.

Stomach

Carnivore's body fluids are acidic so that the digestive fluids can break down raw meat and kill bacteria to process raw meat. Herbivores have alkaline body fluids that aren't meant to digest raw meats.

Think about your own human biology. What group do you belong in? Health reports and our very own physiology prove that human's should follow a vegetarian diet. That's why the whole food plant-based diet is the best lifestyle to follow for good health and longevity.

Grains the Wholesome Way

If you don't normally eat whole grains, now is the time to begin. There are so many health benefits gained from eating whole grain bread, pasta, rice, and cereal that cannot be derived from any processed alternative. Whole grains take the same amount of time to prepare and have not been robbed of all their nutrients like processed foods have.

If it's a matter of taste, you'll find that whole grain alternatives will grow on you. Replace your white bread, white rice, and flour pasta for a whole grain alternative. The refined grains have 90 percent less nutrients than the same whole grain foods. You'd be crazy to not switch over to whole grain knowing that it will improve your health in so many different ways and protect your body.

Whole grains are full of fiber to clean out and maintain a healthy system, complex carbohydrates to fuel your body throughout the day, and tons of other nutrients that fight the risk of many different diseases. Whole grains give you the protein, fiber, vitamins, antioxidants your body needs. On top of that, they are low in saturated fats and lower your risk of cardiovascular disease.

The difference between whole grains and processed foods is that the outer coating, bran, and germ have not been removed in a milling process. When processed foods are milled they leave white flour left over, which doesn't have the same nutritional value whatsoever. Even if the white flour has nutrients added back into it, it still won't compare to the nutritional value of whole grain foods.

American dietary guidelines suggest that you eat 6 to 11 daily servings of grains. You can do this easily since 1 serving isn't much food at all. ½ cup of cooked brown rice, wild rice, sweet potato, barley, quinoa, or oatmeal will do it. ½ of a whole grain bagel is one serving. You can also eat a cup of whole grain cereal, a whole-wheat pancake, one slice of toast, or a cup of buckwheat noodles to add to your intake of grains that are healthy for you.

Vegetables for Promoting Health

Vegetables are another important source of vitamins and minerals that promote positive health. Most people in America don't eat enough servings of vegetables per day and therefore miss out on an opportunity to promote great health and preventing disease.

You can eat vegetables raw, which makes a great snack. You can also cook them minimally to ensure that all of the vitamins and minerals aren't leeched into the water and are retained in your food. Steaming and sautéing are great ways to quickly prepare vegetables in a way that keeps the nutrient value in the vegetables high.

With cruciferous vegetables in your diet, you'll receive a lot of benefits from the phytochemicals that we discussed earlier. These fight cancer, prevent disease, and give us the antioxidants we need to fight free radicals. You'll also benefit from the fiber that's been lacking in your diet if you eat lots of processed foods, in addition to the fact that vegetables are low fat.

If you're losing weight, one great way to do it is by replacing the processed foods in your diet for a serving of vegetables. Your stomach is going to notice all the nutritious food that you're eating and signal to your brain that it's full sooner, and longer. This will cut down on the amount of food you require and give your body the energy that it needs throughout the day.

Eating enough vegetables is very easy to do, especially because one serving of veggies is low, and it's easy to get at least three servings a day. 1 cup of cooked carrots, green beans, spinach, artichoke, or shredded lettuce will add a serving. ½ cup of cooked Brussels sprouts, mushrooms, tomatoes, broccoli, carrots, collard greens, green beans, green peas, lima beans, spinach, or zucchini squash will give you a serving of vegetables.

Replacing just a portion of the meat that you eat daily with a vegetable will do wonders for your health and is easy to do. Find a way to include vegetables with whatever you eat and you'll find yourself exceeding the 5 daily serving requirement easily.

Fruits The Basis of A Plant-based Diet

When people first hear about a whole foods plant-based diet, they immediately jump to the conclusion that they'll only be eating leafy vegetables. Although leafy green veggies are a great source of nutrition, they don't provide the body with everything that it needs to survive. The real basis of a plant-based diet relies on eating enough fruits and starchy plant foods.

Fruits are great sources of nutrients, low in fat and calories, and have plenty of vitamins and fiber. They are a great source of phytochemicals and antioxidants to get rid of the harmful substances in the body that cause disease. Plus there is a wide range of fruits to choose from, each providing your body with different vitamins.

You can easily add fruit to your diet and get the suggested amount of fruits by just replacing any snacks you usually eat with a healthier fruit alternative. One serving of fruit is 1 medium apple, peach, orange, or pear. You can also eat ½ cup of blackberries, blueberries, or raspberries for the same effect. 3 pitted prunes, 4 apricot halves, 6 dates, or 3 tablespoons of raisins are easy to add to your meal, and quickly add a serving of fruit to your diet.

By adding fruit to your diet you not only receive the suggested 2 to 4 daily servings, but you also add the essential vitamins you need to your diet. It isn't difficult to eat extra fruit either, it's all about having it around and available for snacking. Just keep a good selection of fruits with you at your house, and remember to take some with you to work as a great alternative to vending machine food or fast foods.

In the morning you can add fruits to your breakfast foods, or have a bowl of fruit on the side. Pack your lunch full of fruits that you can make into a smoothie or just have separately. Fruit also goes really well with dinner foods, or as an appetizer before the main course. Every meal you should try to add nutrient rich fruits and vegetables to make sure your body is receiving the right amount of nutrients.

When buying fruit at the grocery store, remember to purchase a good variety of fruits. Be open to change and trying new things. You'll not only expand the range of fruits that you enjoy, but you'll also benefit from different vitamins and phytochemicals that help the body fight disease. Here are just a few of the fruits you may want to pick up from the store next time you are doing some shopping:

Apples
Apples are one of the most common types of fruit, with a ton of different varieties. They're a great source of vitamins A, C, K, fiber, sodium, calcium, magnesium, and folic acid. Each apple has around 80 calories.

Apricots
Most apricots are dried or canned. Just 4 halves will provide you with a serving of fruit and gives your body vitamins A, K, fiber, magnesium, calcium and potassium. One serving is about 36 calories altogether.

Bananas
Are you aware that even though it's called a "banana tree" that bananas are really grown on a bush? That makes bananas a herb, and not an actual fruit! Either way, half of a large banana will give you one serving of fruit and provides lots of different vitamins and minerals.

Blueberries
Blueberries are commonly referred to as a superfood because of its rich antioxidant content. Just ½ cup gives you one serving of fruit and provides you with lots of different vitamins and minerals. Eat two servings and you've only consumed 80 calories of delicious blueberries.

Cantaloupe
If you want to fight cancer, cantaloupe is the fruit to eat! It's very rich in carotene, which forms into vitamin A in the body. With only 110 calories in a whole

cantaloupe, you're free to indulge.

Grapes

One cup of grapes gives you vitamins A and C and a range of minerals. At only 90 calories per serving, this is a great food to snack on.

Kiwi

This green fruit is delicious. You can also eat the skin, but many prefer to peel the skin off. However you'd like to eat it, one serving of kiwi gives you lots of vitamins with only 22 calories per oz.

Peaches

Peaches are a great with breakfast cereals and as snacks. One peach is only around 45 calories and full of vitamins A, C, folic acid, potassium and many other great vitamins and minerals.

Pears

Next time you go to the grocery store buy the unripe pears and ripen them in a paper bag at home. This will keep their nutrients locked in, providing you with tons of vitamins and minerals when it's time for a snack. A pear will fill you up too since it provides 100 calories for fueling your body.

Pineapple

Pineapple is juicy, sweet, and gives your body just 75 calories per cup of fruit. In addition to being low in calories, it also has the power to aid digestion and help recover from cardiovascular disease.

Plums

This tart fruit was one of the first in human civilization to be domesticated. At only 32 calories don't be afraid to eat a couple. It gives your body vitamin A, C, fiber, and potassium.

Raisins

Just a handful of raisins gives you vitamins A, C, folic acid, and potassium. It's high in sugar, so they'll also give you lots of extra energy.

Raspberries

Just a half cup of raspberries will give you lots of great vitamins and minerals with only 30 calories. They go bad fairly quickly so make sure that you add it to cereals and use them for a snack. There are hundreds of different varieties of raspberry found throughout the world.

Watermelon
Watermelon is low in calories with only 50 calories per cup. It's also very nutrient rich. You can get it seedless or with seeds, and even in a square shape in Japan and other Asian countries.

Legumes, Nuts, and Seeds

If you are looking for a great way to boost the amount of protein that you receive on the whole foods plant-based diet, consider eating more legumes, nuts, and seeds. Not only are these foods filled with lots of great proteins, but they also are low in fat and sodium. They also provide you with high levels of fiber, vitamins, and minerals.

Legumes include beans, peas, and lentils. These foods provide us with lasting energy throughout the day, lower cholesterol in the blood, and are inexpensive compared to animal products. You can add legumes to lots of different dishes and receive the rich nutrients that they offer to your diet.

Nuts and seeds are also a great source of protein. You'll also benefit from high levels of good fats, high fiber levels and a ton of vitamins. Eating a diet rich in nuts and seeds can reduce your risk of developing cardiovascular disease, making it less likely for blood to clot in your body thanks to production of special amino acids.

Nuts and seeds have high fat contents. Fortunately nuts are low in saturated fat and high in monounsaturated and polyunsaturated fat. This will help prevent cardiovascular disease and reduce the amount of bad cholesterol that is located in your body. Make sure that the nuts you eat are raw and have no salt added, so that you do not undermine the positive health benefits. There are also some varieties of nuts that are high in saturated fat such as Brazil nuts, macadamia nuts, and cashews that you should eat sparingly.

If you are trying to limit the amount of fat you have in your diet, just use nuts and seeds as a light snack. Eat them in moderation for the nutrients they contain, and add them to cereals, and other dishes.

Legumes are going to be a main way to receive the proper amounts of protein in your diet. There are many different varieties of legumes to choose from, and they are easily added to foods or eaten alone as snacks. If you purchase the precooked cans, make sure that no sodium has been added already. If you have extra time, you can also prepare dry beans yourself, but it requires a good 2 – 3 hours or longer to soak the beans.

Keep a range of legumes, nuts, and seeds available to eat every day to ensure that you get a wide range of protein types. The best way to make sure you get enough protein is by eating a range of foods each day. If you eat legumes, nuts, or seeds, a whole grain, and fruits and vegetables, you'll guarantee that your body can form complete proteins in your body.

Foods to Increase Your Protein Levels

Most people in the Western world don't face a protein deficiency since protein is usually the main course of a meal. The issue is finding alternative protein sources of foods that aren't high in fat, and that don't contribute to high cholesterol levels, but rather make you healthier and lower your amount of cholesterol.

On a whole foods plant-based diet you receive all of your protein from plant-based foods instead of from animal proteins, fish, or other animal products. The great thing about protein is that it's naturally found in plant-based foods. Legumes have plenty of protein without the high levels of sodium, saturated fat, and cholesterol.

Nuts and seeds also give you plenty of proteins. You not only receive protein by eating plant-based foods, but you also get a ton of vitamins, minerals, and a mixture of your healthy fats. You receive lots of fiber by eating plant-based proteins, which clean out your system, reduce cholesterol levels, and prevent constipation.

With a plant-based food diet you really don't have to worry about getting enough protein for your body. As long as you are eating enough calories from a variety of plant based foods there's no way that you can be deficient in protein. In fact you'll consume proteins at a much healthier level that promotes positive health.

Depending on your level of activity and body weight, you may require more or less protein than people in your age range. You likely need somewhere between 40 – 60 grams of protein per day, which is most likely a lot less than you're actually getting. Excess protein is either used as energy in the body and doesn't contribute to muscle mass, or is turned into fat, so there really isn't a need to eat more than the required amount of protein in your diet. Excess protein in the diet has also been linked to kidney disease, calcium stones in the kidney, and osteoporosis.

There's a good mix of protein in just about everything you'll be eating throughout the day on a whole foods plant-based diet. If you're worried about not getting enough, all you have to do is add a small amount of legumes, nuts, fruits, and vegetables to your diet and it'll be easy to ensure that you get your daily requirement of protein.

The Empty Calorie Issue

At the top of the food pyramid you have foods that are high in fat and high in calories. These foods really don't provide you with any nutrients and are unhealthy due to their fat, sugar, and salt contents which all increase your risk of cardiovascular disease.

Many of these foods are known as providing empty calories because they lack nutritional value, so eating them as the primary foods in your diet can result in getting enough calories but being malnourished. Foods with high fat content and high sugar content should be avoided on the whole foods plant-based diet.

Examples of empty calorie foods include soda, cakes and pies, milkshakes, cookies, chips, jellybeans, ice cream, and popcorn that's cooked in oil. Removing empty calories from your diet and replacing it with healthier alternatives like fruit can cure your sweet tooth but more importantly provide your body nutrients and minimize the risk of disease.

Everything Your Need To Know About Weight Control

The Importance of Weight Control

Some of you who are going to start a whole foods plant-based diet are doing so that you can easily manage your weight. That's a very great reason to start this diet, and hopefully the changes that you experience with this diet helps you continue this lifestyle even after the weight is off.

There are a number of reasons that one would go on a diet with the most important being the health benefit that you'll experience. Getting to a average weight for your height is very important and lowers your risk of having high blood pressure, high cholesterol, developing cardiovascular disease, diabetes, and so much more.

Excess weight puts a lot of stress on your heart, bones, and muscles. Just a small reduction in your weight can really start the process of creating a more healthy and energetic you. Plus you'll lower your risk of a premature death, and greatly lower your risk of preventable disease.

In addition to the health benefits, you'll also improve your appearance, have a higher self-esteem, and feel a lot better mentally and emotionally. To control your weight, you need to adopt life-long changes and not just follow a fad diet that you'll quit in a couple months.

How The Whole Foods Plant-Based Diet Helps Your Lose Weight

A whole foods plant-based diet can be the lifestyle change you need. Eating whole foods in addition to being active can help you shed the pounds for good. You'll eat until you're full and never feel hungry, you'll enjoy eating the foods you love, and you'll notice that you feel full a lot sooner since the food provides you more energy throughout the day.

What's wonderful about the whole foods plant-based diet is that it follows all the rules that allow you to easily control and maintain your weight. You can eat foods until you're full. You'll eat exactly what you need, cutting out the fat and junk foods and replacing them with healthy fruits and vegetables. These changes will bring about revitalization and fight fatigue throughout the day.

A lot of times, people hate having restrictions on them that says you can only eat so much of this, or so much of that. Instead of limiting you like that, you can still eat the foods that you enjoy. Instead of saying you should only get a certain amount of calories per day, you're free to eat until you're full.

The difference is that you'll eat a variety of foods with a high calorie density. That means the calories per pound will give your body everything that it needs while also feeling full afterward. Your stomach will tell your brain, "I've gotten enough food," because it will be nutritious and won't just provide you with a little energy that quickly fades away; instead it will give you the fuel necessary to get through the day.

On a plant-based diet you don't have the oil, the sugars, or the meat to add extra fat to your diet. These foods are overly calorie dense. By basing your diet around them you make it so that your stomach doesn't think that it's getting a large enough of those foods - even though you're getting way more than necessary. All the food that would just add to your midsection and cause health problems is totally eliminated from your diet.

Instead you'll eat fruits, vegetables, legumes, whole grains, and healthy starchy foods. You'll supercharge the amount of nutrients your body is receiving from all of your food, and you'll notice the benefits in your health. Your food will fill you up and your body won't need additional fuel just to get you through the day. Continue with the diet and the weight loss and health benefits will be tremendous.

Goal Setting and Weight Loss

When it comes to setting weight loss goals, it's important to not push yourself too much at the beginning, and to maintain a diet that is healthy and you can follow for a long time. The whole foods plant-based diet really shouldn't be called a diet. It's really more of a lifestyle change because the benefits are so great that the diet is easily maintained, and you really won't want to switch back to an animal-based diet.

So first, start with a realistic goal for losing weight. At the beginning a safe amount of weight loss is about one percent of your body weight per week. Remember that dieting is a gradual change, one that takes time. Aiming for a smaller amount of weight loss insures that you are staying healthy and not losing muscle or fluid. Instead you want to target the fat and remain healthy.

With a whole foods plant-based diet you'll notice health improvements in areas other than your weight alone. You'll feel more active, you'll reduce your amount of cholesterol in the blood, and might even notice that some of the symptoms of any issues you have reduced or even been eliminated.

Even if the weight loss isn't occurring as rapidly as you would like, don't give up! There are many other benefits to eating healthy and staying active.

So what is required in a standard diet to promote weight loss? Let's break it down right here:

3 – 5 Servings of Vegetables I guarantee you that you'll eat more than that on a whole foods plant-based diet. Any time you can add a serving of vegetables to your meal, you should. This will make you feel full faster since most vegetables have a low calorie density, and they'll add lots of great nutrients to your diet. You can have your starchy vegetables here, which will be one main area of your diet.

2 – 4 Servings of Fruit You'll probably exceed this amount too, and that's wonderful. You already know about the phytochemicals that are in fruits and vegetables. In order to get them, eat a range of fruits throughout the day. They'll give you lots of lasting energy and work

great when you want to snack. It's easy to add fruits to breakfast, lunch, and dinner by adding it to your foods, having it on the side, or drinking a smoothie or fruit juice.

6 Servings of Breads and Cereals

This is where the whole grains come in. Add some to breakfast, lunch, and dinner and you'll get a nice mix of the foods that you need throughout the day. It's the overall picture of the food you're eating that promotes health. By choosing whole grain foods to add to your diet you're getting all of the health benefits from whole grains, filling your stomach with the right foods, and adding protein to your meals.

2 – 3 Servings of Protein

All of the proteins that you eat will be low fat, low sodium, and low cholesterol. Just a half-cup of the right legumes can give you one serving of the protein you need through the day.

Combine it with the other foods that you have been eating and you'll never have to worry about not getting enough protein in your diet. Plant-based protein sources are heart healthy and will help you lose weight.

With a whole foods plant-based diet you'll get all of the adequate required servings of foods to help you lose weight. With this combination of foods you increase the amount of nutrients that you receive from your food and forgo all of the fat, sugars, and foods that cause disease.

How The Body Tells You That You're Full

As you change your standard diet and start supplying your body with foods that are nutrient and vitamin rich, your stomach will notice the difference. The full feeling that you get after eating isn't actually the result of too much food being in your stomach. In fact it's a chemical response triggered by your stomach that happens in your brain to inform you that you've had enough.

Losing weight with the whole foods plant-based diet is easy because you're giving yourself nutrient rich food isn't calorie dense. Even though oil and meat gives you a lot of calories per serving, you don't normally feel satisfied with just a steak. That's because foods that are high in fat don't signal to your brain that you've received enough food as soon which causes you to overeat.

Foods that are high in fiber, protein, and water such as your fruits, vegetables, and starchy foods signal to your brain that you're full and in turn you feel satisfied on fewer calories. On a whole foods plant-based diet you'll receive the exact nutrients that your body needs at levels that will help you maintain a healthy weight.

Adding Regular Exercise

The foods that you eat give you the energy to engage in physical exercise. When you fail to exercise enough and exert the energy you have then your body weight increases. Physical activity during the weight loss process is just as important as eating is. If you aren't planning to increase your level of activity, don't use that as a reason to not begin a whole foods plant-based diet. Just improving your diet is more helpful than making no life changes.

If it has been a while since you last had a regular exercise routine, make sure that you start slowly. Begin by walking and overtime you can increase your effort. If you start too extreme with your exercise routine you'll risk injuring your body, which will only cause you to stop exercising altogether.

Just like with a diet, you also want to incorporate exercise that is at a good level for you. It's good to have both an anaerobic and aerobic exercise plan. Anaerobic exercises build your strength through resistance training like lifting weights. Aerobic exercise increases your heart rate and burns fat. This includes running, swimming, and dancing.

Always check with your doctor before beginning an exercise routine. You want to make sure that your heart can handle the stress of a workout before doing anything too strenuous. Your level of activity doesn't have to be rigorous and can be as simple as cleaning your home, gardening, or washing the car.

You also have the option of talking to a fitness professional to have them assist you with a personalized routine that will work with your goals. They can help keep you motivated and accountable. It's always good to have a support system while you are trying to achieve any goal, and finding a fitness partner will also push you to lose weight and become healthy.

There are many benefits to promoting health through exercise. You can lower your blood pressure, lose or maintain your weight, and increase your muscle strength. When mixed with a whole foods plant-based diet, you'll notice changes in the amount of energy you have and feel great.

Food As Medicine

Improving Your Health

The food you eat and the nutrients you supply your body have the biggest effect on your health. By eating the right foods and maintaining the proper diet, you can ensure health throughout your years. If you suffer from any diseases or health problems, it's not too late to adopt good eating habits and reverse the disease altogether.

Taking medication doesn't get to the root of a health problem. It only treats the symptoms and not always the underlying problems. Occasionally it even creates new problems in the body that then has to be treated with more medications. It doesn't have to be this way. You can allow your body to heal itself by eating the right foods.

It's possible that a healthy whole foods plant-based diet can help you remove yourself from your medications. You'll notice that once you change your diet and adopt a whole foods plant-based lifestyle that some of your symptoms will disappear, and you may require a lower dose of your medication, or downright be able to stop taking it altogether.

When you begin feeling healthier, stronger, and notice common problems that you've taken medication to solve for years, talk to your doctor about the changes brought about by your diet and see what's recommended in your case.

When you stop adopting the diet of the Western world that's full of unnecessary fats, an abundance of salt, and foods that cause disease, you'll notice immediate improvements to your health. You'll lower your risk of cancer, cardiovascular disease, diabetes, and osteoporosis.

With a whole foods plant-based diet you'll transition from the foods that create health problems and start eating the foods that cure them. You won't rely on fatty or processed foods in your diet, and you'll begin to feel improvements in your level of energy.

What you eat and drink is what you become. Do you want to be full of vital nutrients that bring about longevity or would you rather crash like a sugar rush? Hopefully the choice is obvious and you begin eating the right foods to improve your health today. Lets start by discussing how you can figure out how much nutrients is in the food that you purchase from the grocery store.

Reading The Food Labels

Ideally you should stock your kitchen and pantry with foods that don't have labels, but there are a few different types of food out there that have been packaged and are still healthy for you.

The important thing to note is that you can't really trust the front of the container. You have to flip it around and look at the specific details about the food you're thinking about buying.

You should see the front package as marketing. Businesses will do whatever they need to for you to pick up the package and purchase it. Sometimes there will only be a small fact or two about the nutrients found in the package without giving you a clear picture of if the food is actually healthy.

Here are the five main questions to ask yourself while reviewing a label:

What are the ingredients? You want to find products with whole grains at the top of the list, with the actual grain type listed.

What is the serving size? Some companies will list low serving sizes to make it seem like their product is healthier than it is. Ask yourself whether you are going to really eat the food following that serving size and if not, review what the actual nutrients in the product actually are.

How much fat is in this food? Ideally you want the fat in your food to be under 15%. If the food provides less than 15 calories of fat for every 100 calories, then the food meets the fat criteria.

How much sodium is in this food? Keep the sodium to 1mg per calorie unless you're only using a small portion of the food.

How much sugar has been added? Look for all the varieties of sugar on the label, not just for the word sugar. Since the nutrients on the label are listed depending on how much of it are found in the product, look for products that list only one form of sugar that is listed low on the list. You should avoid any products with sugar as one of the main nutrients.

Once a food follows all of those requirements, it has passed the test! Now you know exactly what to look for in the foods you purchase, and what are good indications that the food is actually as healthy as it seems.

Superfoods

Green foods provide you with lots of vitamins and minerals to stay healthy. There are some foods that are green and considered superfoods too! Here's a list of foods that are considered superfoods and their benefits. Add them to your diet to boost how you feel each day.

Grasses like wheat grass and barley grass promote healthy blood, are super packed with calcium, vitamin C, and other nutrients.

Spirulina is an algae that is packed with tons of protein, can help you lose weight, and even controls blood sugar levels.

Blueberries activate fat fighting cells, provide a high level of antioxidants, and improve the body's ability to fight off infection.

Broccoli is one of the best superfoods for fighting cancer and other diseases. It has high levels of vitamin C, beta-carotene and other nutrients.

Flaxseed provides your body with omega-3 fatty acid that helps your heart. It's also rich in fiber and phytonutrients.

Legumes are rich in fiber, protein, folic acid and many other nutrients. Legumes can help replace red meats in your diet, and lower the level of cholesterol in your blood.

Nuts are rich in healthy plant fats that lower cholesterol and packed with tons of nutrients such as selenium and vitamin E.

Oatmeal is loaded with great levels of fiber and keep you feeling full longer. It slows your metabolism, prevents heart disease, and lowers blood cholesterol levels.

Oranges nearly give you your required amount of vitamin C in one serving. It's great for your immune system, helps fight off cancers and protects against cardiovascular disease.

Peppers are great for eyesight, maybe even better than carrots! It's a great source of vitamin C and beta-carotene. These antioxidants fight free radicals to ward disease. Lycopene is what gives certain peppers their red color, which has been tested to ward off lung and prostate cancer.

Quinoa is a very nutritious grain that is high in protein, manganese, iron, and even has small amounts of omega-3 fatty acids. It's also gluten free and one of the first crops that NASA is thinking about planting in outer space.

Red Grapes are rich in phytonutrients and abundant in places throughout the world. It's also antioxidant rich and has been proven to protect against cancer.

Spinach has antioxidant properties and provides the body with a lot of great energy. It contains a lot of great nutrients like iron, protein, and vitamins K, A, and C. Since spinach has high water content, it reduces greatly once cooked. Be liberal when cooking it as it only contains 23 calories per 100 grams.

Tomatoes provide the antioxidant lycopene, which is rarely found in other foods. Tomatoes fight against certain types of cancer, have high amounts of vitamins and minerals and even protect the body against harmful UV rays.

Most **green leafy vegetables** are also considered superfoods because they lower the risk of cancer and heart disease.

They help the brain, immune system, and kidneys and act as a body cleanser.

Reducing Cardiovascular Disease Risks

Cardiovascular disease includes a number of disorders including heart attach, stroke, high blood cholesterol, and high blood pressure. All of these problems put stress on your heart and arteries. If you suffer from any of these problems you can treat and prevent them by following a healthy diet.

The saturated fat, trans fat, and cholesterol in your diet play a huge role in the amount of cholesterol that is in your blood. Eventually these dietary problems lead to a heart attack or stroke. By cutting out the fats and foods that are high in cholesterol, you can begin to repair your body.

One way to stop eating foods that are high in fat is to replace them with fruits, vegetables, and legumes.

You can still get all of the nutrients that you need in your diet – including protein – at much healthier levels that are good for your heart and your arteries. Switching from processed foods to whole grains are also very heart healthy and can help prevent angina, coronary heart disease, high blood pressure, and many other cardiovascular diseases.

Following a whole foods plant-based lifestyle will help decrease the bad cholesterol in your body, decrease triglyceride levels in your body, and raise the amount of good cholesterol in your blood. It's been proven that there's a link between diet and cardiovascular disease. Following a plant-based diet is the easiest way to repair your body and give it the proper nutrients that it needs to thrive.

Reducing Your Risk For Respiratory Disorders

Just like with cardiovascular disease, you can treat and prevent respiratory disorders with the proper diet. Any disorder that blocks the passage of air through our system is a respiratory disorder, with the most common ones being chronic obstructive pulmonary disease, sleep apnea, and asthma.

Chronic obstructive pulmonary disease is the effect of two different conditions of the respiratory disorder, bronchitis and emphysema. Damage occurs in the lungs making it harder to breath normally. This damage is usually irreversible, and can cause weight loss, since it is also difficult to eat.

With COPD, weight loss can make breathing worse, which is why it's important to stay on a proper diet to avoid undernutrition. A diet full of the essential vitamins, minerals, and antioxidants is key to protect against COPD and increase the strength of people who are suffering from COPD. If you suffer from COPD and undernutrition, you should eat healthy high calorie foods that aren't fatty and give the body lots of nutrients.

If you suffer from sleep apnea, one of the best ways to reduce the symptoms includes losing and maintaining the proper weight. It's important to get help from a doctor when it comes to losing weight while suffering from sleep apnea.

Some changes that you should make to promote weight loss are to snack on low fat, nutrient rich foods like fruits and vegetables instead of on foods that are high in fat, salt, or sugar. Control your portion sizes and limit your caloric intake. Also avoid empty calories from alcohol, which may only worsen the conditions of sleep apnea.

Those who suffer from asthma often have increased dietary needs, especially if using an inhaler to send corticosteroids to the lungs.

This can put excess stress on the body and require that you receive more vitamins and minerals in your diet.

Asthmatics have different foods that trigger asthma symptoms in the body. It's important to avoid those triggers and to eat a diet that is balanced and nutritious to improve asthma symptoms. Foods such as dairy products, meat, fish, citrus, wheat, and soy are common triggers.

A whole food plant-based diet is a great option for someone who suffers from any of these respiratory disorders and wants to reduce their symptoms through a good diet. You'll get all of the nutrients that you need in abundance, and it can help you lose weight, stay fully nourished, and reduce symptoms that are caused by these disorders.

Eating Right for Digestive Disorders

The digestive process begins when you put food in your

mouth and ends when your body releases the waste that's leftover. In between those two processes, food makes its way through a long track in the body that breaks down food, removes the nutrients required by your body and sends them to the correct places. Those nutrients are used for energy, growth, and repair of the body.

When something goes wrong during this process, a digestive disorder begins. Most are short term like diarrhea, constipation, and indigestion. Some are long-term and are caused by specific foods in the diet. Following the proper diet and making the necessary lifestyle changes can treat all of the problems that come about from digestive disorders.

Lets discuss each disorder and what you can do to help the problem:

Indigestion causes pain in the abdomen after eating. You can avoid this by eating foods that don't cause indigestion. Usually spicy and acidic foods cause indigestion. Instead eat smaller portions that don't cause discomfort and are low in fat.

Constipation causes your body to have a difficult time releasing waste. You can relieve this by eating food that is rich in fiber, and by drinking water.

Diarrhea causes your body to have stool that is too watery and loose. To reduce the symptoms of diarrhea, make sure that you understand the problem that is causing it. Sometimes this can be an infection. If it's a short-term problem then avoid foods with fiber for a short time. If it is persistent diarrhea then increase your fiber intake.

Irritable bowl syndrome causes pain, gas, and excess bowel movements. Adopt a diet full of low fat and fiber rich foods.

Gastroesophageal reflux disease is caused by acid regurgitating in the esophagus and causes chest pain. Symptoms can be reduced by losing weight and by following a low fat and fiber rich diet.

Peptic ulcers are caused by damage of the stomach and small intestine. Reduce the ulcers by reducing the amount of alcohol, caffeine, and spicy foods in the diet. Quitting smoking also helps.

Lactose intolerance stops the sufferer from being able to consume sugars known as lactose. Avoiding dairy products and consuming lactose free drinks helps this problem.

Celiac disease stops people from being able to absorb gluten products. You can avoid gluten foods to stop any damage in your small intestine from occurring.

Crohn's disease is an inflammatory disorder of the ileum and colon. Avoid this by following a low fat, low fiber, and low lactose diet.

Ulcerative colitis causes ulcers that affect the colon. Reduce the symptoms by eating foods rich in fiber and by taking vitamin supplements.

Diverticular disease causes pouches in the colon that are painful and may become inflamed. Reduce these problems by drinking lots of water daily and by eating foods rich in fiber.

Many of the different digestive disorders can be solved with a good diet that is rich in fiber, and low fat. Adopting a whole foods plant-based lifestyle is a great choice for you if you suffer from any of these disorders, as it will help you body recover from the problems that you face daily.

Reducing Bone and Joint Disorders Through Food

Keeping your bones healthy throughout life is a matter of getting the proper nutrition and exercise. The bones work with your muscles to help you stay mobile. There are many different bone and joint disorders that occur when someone makes poor diet and lifestyle decisions.

The most common bone and joint disorders are osteoporosis, osteomalacia, and arthritis. These problems are avoided with the proper diet and the symptoms of these disorders can also be maintained by introducing nutrient rich foods in your diet.

To reduce the chance of developing osteoporosis, which occurs when the bones lose important bone tissue that increases the risk of fracture, you should get enough calcium in your diet. Calcium isn't produced within your body, but it's used to strengthen bones and teeth and for other processed. If your body requires additional calcium then it won't continue to supply an adequate amount of calcium to the bones and instead will take away from your bone structure.

You should also increase your intake of vitamin D, which helps with the absorption of calcium. It's common for those who lack the proper amount of vitamin D to also have problems with bone density. This places them at greater risk for any bone and joint disorder. Another important factor is getting the correct amount of exercise. Exercise increases bone mass and reduces the amount of bone loss that occurs with osteoporosis.

Cutting back on acidic foods will greatly reduce your risk of bone disease. Acidic foods slowly break down the calcium in your bones and stop the natural absorption of calcium from occurring. You should avoid milk, white grains, and sugars to ensure that your diet is low in acid-forming foods.

Some other factors that increase your risk of osteoporosis include smoking, overconsumption of alcohol, and low amounts of physical activity. By reducing the amount of alcohol you consume, quitting smoking, and getting the proper amount of exercise you can greatly reduce your risk of having osteoporosis.

Osteomalacia is similar to osteoporosis where as it has to do with you body not properly absorbing calcium. Vitamin D deficiency also comes into play here, as do disorders in the absorption process of foods in the intestine such as Celiac disease.

Osteomalacia is characterized by soft bones and can also be caused by a lack of sunlight. It leads to pain in throughout the body in the muscles and at the joints. Since the bones have been softened, it becomes very easily to break the bones in your body, which impair mobility.

Osteomalacia also occurs in children, where it's known as rickets. Rickets is most common with babies who are breast fed without getting enough vitamin D, especially those that don't get enough exposure to sunlight. Most children however do not develop rickets since vitamin D is fortified in milk.

Vitamin D comes from two sources. Exposure to sunlight helps your body create the vitamin D that you need. You can also receive it from foods which is especially important if you live somewhere that lacks in sunlight for part of the year, or if you don't get outside much. Still you can't receive all of the vitamin D from the sun, which makes it necessary to eat a wide variety of food or take a supplement.

If you follow a plant-based diet and are wondering what you should consume to ensure that you have enough vitamin D in your diet, all you have to do is find a plant-based milk that is fortified with vitamin D. If you don't drink plant milk often then taking a vitamin supplement may be necessary depending on your level of outdoor activity.

Another major bone and joint disorder in the Western world is arthritis. There are many different arthritic conditions that cause pain and stiffness in the joints. Rheumatoid arthritis, osteoarthritis, and gout are common forms of arthritis that can affect various areas of the body.

It's recommended that you receive about 1000 – 1200mg of calcium per day depending on your age. So what foods can you eat to increase your level of dietary calcium without eating animal products? Here's a list of foods that are full of calcium:

Adzuki Beans
Almond Butter
Amaranth
Artichoke
Black Currants
Blackberries
Blackstrap Molasses
Broccoli
Collard Greens
Fortified Non-Dairy Milk
Fortified Orange Juice
Great Northern Beans
Hemp Milk
Kale
Navy Beans
Oranges
Raw Fennel
Sesame Seeds
Soybeans
Tahini
Tempeh
Turnip Greens

What's great about these sources of calcium is that they will keep your levels of cholesterol down, are full of fiber, vitamins, and minerals. With all these options and more, it's easy for anyone who is following a plant-based diet to make sure that they receive enough calcium.

In addition to consuming enough calcium, you should also have a proper nutrient rich diet if you suffer from arthritis. One of the symptoms of rheumatoid arthritis is that your joints suffer from inflammation, which causes swelling and pain. Medications that are anti-inflammatory might reduce the amount that nutrients are absorbed in the body, calling for a nutrient rich diet to ensure that you don't become deficient.

You'll want to increase your intake of foods that are rich in vitamins E, B and D, as well as calcium, iron, omega-3 fatty acids, and antioxidants. Each of these help your bones and joints function normally and can reduce the amount of pain that is caused by arthritis.

Overall your diet may not be able to totally cure all of the different types of bone and joint disorders, but it does affect the severity of the symptoms and guarantees that you are receiving the proper nutrients for good health. Certain vitamins and minerals like calcium and vitamin D are definitely able to counteract bone loss and can help your body remain strong. Mix a solid plant-based diet with enough exercise and you should be able to lessen the effects of joint and bone disorders.

How Your Diet Effects Diabetes

Many people throughout the United States have diabetes, and many more have prediabetes. As the number of people who are obese rises, so do the number of people who develop a problem with high blood glucose levels. Type 2 diabetes is preventable and that portion accounts for nearly 95% of all diagnosed cases of diabetes. There's also a little data that type 1 diabetes is triggered in some cases due to the diet of people who are genetically predisposed to diabetes.

Diabetes occurs when glucose in the blood is at a very high level. Glucose is the main sugar that is converted from carbohydrates to be used as energy. In order for glucose to enter body cells the hormone insulin has to be produced within the body. Without enough insulin, the glucose stays in the bloodstream and doesn't get converted to energy. Diabetic treatments try to solve the problem of restoring the amount of insulin that's in the body to the proper levels.

Type 1 diabetes is the less common form of diabetes that occurs in children and people under the age of 30. There is some evidence that reducing your amount of dairy can potentially reduce the risk of type 1 diabetes and cancer. Type 1 diabetes is a result of insulin producing cells in the pancreas being damaged or destroyed to the point where insulin in no longer produced. Without the correct amount of insulin in the body, ketoacidosis can occur.

The body giving up on using carbohydrates for energy and instead breaking down fats as a source of energy instead causes Ketoacidosis. The breakdown of fats leaves a chemical called ketones in the body that causes weakness, fatigue, dehydration, coma, and even death if the level of ketones gets too high.

Type 2 diabetes on the other hand begins as prediabetes and develops if changes in lifestyle and diet don't occur. Prediabetes occurs when the insulin in the body either isn't used properly to assist glucose into forming energy, or if the body doesn't produce enough insulin. Diet plays a big role in insulin resistance and can delay or even prevent type 2 diabetes.

Unlike type 1 diabetes, people who develop type 2 diabetes don't require insulin within the first few years of it's development since their body still produces it. Instead the glucose in their body continues to rise if the proper lifestyle and diet changes aren't made, which brings about the same symptoms that occur in type 1 diabetics such as excessive hunger, lack of energy, vomiting, and nausea.

If you have diabetes, don't worry that you won't be able to eat sugars or carbs. It just means that you have to make sure that your diet consists of the proper level of nutrients that your body needs. A whole foods plant-based diet is a great diet for you to consider because it reduces your dietary fat and consumption of dairy products to cut your calories and help you lose weight to better manage your diabetes. This is especially important for people who have developed type 2 diabetes.

People with both type 1 and type 2 diabetes should focus on eating carbohydrates that have low glycemic-index values, which take longer to break down in the body and provide glucose steadily, instead of raising blood sugar levels too rapidly. Many of the carbohydrates that you eat on a plant-based diet have a low glycemic-index value including oats and whole grain pasta.

If you are diabetic and interested in promoting your health through healthy eating practices, a whole foods plant-based diet can definitely give you the nutrients you need and support your dietary restrictions. For prediabetics, it could slow down the transition into type 2 diabetes or even stop it from occurring altogether.

For those of you who do have type 2 diabetes, it a plant-based diet can help you lose weight, manage your blood sugar levels, and lower your blood cholesterol and triglyceride levels. It's recommended that you consider making the change for your health and well-being.

Eating To Reduce the Risk of Cancer

Cancer occurs when abnormal cells grow and spread throughout the body. It commonly starts as tumors in the breast, skin, lung, intestine, or prostate. From there it travels through blood and glands to other areas. Statistically, half of the men living and a third of women living in America will develop cancer at some point during their lifetime. Lifestyle changes including your diet can help prevent and treat cancer.

Diet most commonly influences cancer of the breast, prostate, and colon. You can reduce your risk of developing these cancers by maintaining a diet that is full of the nutrients your body needs. Lets discuss the facts about cancer and nutrition, and what changes you can make in your diet to prevent the cancer:

Eat Plenty of Fruits and Vegetables
Fruits and vegetables give you plenty of vitamins, minerals, phytochemicals, and fiber. Many different varieties of fruits and vegetables have been proven to fight disease, including cancer.

Reduce Your Fat Intake
When you eat an excess amount of fat and calories that your body doesn't require, you end up gaining weight. People that are overweight or obese are at greater risk for some forms of cancer. For this reason it's important that your diet is low fat. You should reduce the amount of meats you eat, as well as foods that are high in fat, and foods that have a high calorie density. Opt for healthier low fat options, and reduce your weight to reduce your risk of cancer.

Get Plenty of Fiber
Fiber works like an antioxidant to fight off free radicals in the body that can promote the growth of cancer cells. You can get plenty of fiber from plant-based sources such as whole

grains, fruits, and vegetables. In addition, whole grains, fruits, and vegetables give you lots of other vitamins and minerals and provide you with extra antioxidants to fight cancer.

Lose Weight: With a plant-based diet you can eat all the foods you want until you're full and still lose weight. This is because your body realizes that you have the proper level of nutrients in your food and because you are filling your stomach with foods that are low density and nutritious. Losing extra weight greatly reduces your risk for cancer and brings about a lot of other positive health changes as well. By following a plant-based diet you won't only lose the weight, but you'll keep it off as well.

The best foods that are known to fight cancer are all plant-based foods. You won't find dairy products or animal products on the list of best foods to eat while fighting cancer, but you will find fruits, vegetables, legumes, and whole grains. Let's discuss which foods you should eat while going through cancer treatment:

Cruciferous Vegetables: Broccoli, cauliflower, brussels sprouts, and other similar vegetables help increase antioxidant levels in the body that are used to fight cancer cells.

Nuts and Seeds: These are full of good fats, phenolic acid, and selenium, which can help fight cancer of the prostate.

Green and Black Tea: Teas contain flavonoids and polyphenols that can protect you against stomach cancer.

Orange Fruits and Vegetables: Carotenoids and beta-carotene gives the vegetables their orange color and contain antioxidants to fight off cancer.

Whole Grains: Whole grains are great

sources of fiber that helps regulate the system and flush it out to reduce the risk of cancer.

Cancer can be prevented and aid the curing process if you get the right nutrients in your diet. A whole foods plant-based diet might be the solution you are looking for. It's filled with tons of healthy foods that help reduce the risk of cancer, and fight it altogether. It's vital that you fill you body with food that will aid in its recovery and plant-based foods do just that.

A Whole Food Plant-Based Shopping List

Getting Rid of Your Existing Foods

Review the section on reading the food labels and remind yourself of the questions that you should ask about any food that you want to include in your diet. Use those same criteria against the food in your household.

Remember that you can do this gradually and ease into your new diet if you wish. You have the freedom to begin with breakfast and purchase the foods you need to have your first meal of the day be a whole foods plant-based meal. Once you are used to it, you can stock your house with lunch foods, and then dinner foods.

Sometimes it's easier to just jump into the change rapidly once you've exhausted your food reservoirs. If you want you can purchase everything you need for breakfast, lunch, and dinner the whole foods plant-based way. It's up to you how you'd like to do it.

When you have decided what you'd like to do, go ahead and get rid of the foods that no longer fit in with your existing diet. If any of the food you normally eat is too high in fat, sugar, salt, or includes ingredients that you won't be eating anymore, then donate the food to a food bank or give it to your neighbor.

Once your shelves are empty you'll be ready to stock everything up again with nutritious plant-based foods.

What to Stock Your Kitchen With

When you stock your kitchen, make sure to purchase the foods that you love to eat that follow the diet and are oil free. If there is a low fat or low sodium variety available, opt for those instead. The more healthy options that you have in your refrigerator and pantry, the easier it will be to follow this diet and gain benefits from the foods that you eat. Below is a list of foods that you should purchase. You only need to have a few from each category.

Sauces and Dips – Tahini, Ketchup, Mustard, Sriracha, Harissa, BBQ Sauce, Pesto, Teriyaki, Soy Sauce or Tamari Sauce, Hoisin Sauce, Sofrito, Salsa, Satay Sauce

Low Sugar Jelly or Jam – Apricot, Grape, Strawberry, Raspberry, Orange

Plant Based Milk – Soy Milk, Hemp Milk, Almond Milk, Hazelnut Milk, Oat Milk, Rice Milk

Fresh Fruits and Frozen Fruits – Apples, Apricot, Blackberries, Blueberries, Dates, Figs, Peach, Orange, Pear, Prunes, Raisins, Raspberries, Strawberries, Lemon, Lime

Dried Fruit – Apple, Mango, Apricot, Cherry, Fig, Papaya, Blueberries, Raisins, Black Currant, Plum, Pear, Tomato

Fresh Vegetables and Frozen Vegetables – Artichoke, Broccoli, Brussels Sprouts, Carrots, Collard Greens, Green Peas, Lima Beans, Spinach, Zucchini Squash, Onions, Garlic, Ginger

Canned Vegetables

Vegetable Broth

Canned Tomatoes

Frozen Cooked Grains – Black Barley, Brown Rice, Wheat Berries, Brown Rice (you can also cook and freeze grains yourself!)

Potatoes – Sweet Potatoes, Russet Potatoes, Red Potatoes, White Potatoes, Yellow Potatoes, Purple Potatoes, Fingerling Potatoes, Petite Potatoes

Grains – Whole Wheat, Whole Oats, Bulgur, Brown Rice, Barley, Whole Rye, Buckwheat, Couscous, Quinoa, Freekeh

Corn or Wheat Tortillas

Cornmeal

Baked Tortilla Chips

Whole Grain Pasta

Tomato Sauce and Paste (with nothing added)

Pasta Sauce

Whole Grain Pizza Crust

Cold Cereals and Oatmeal

Beans (Dry and canned with no sodium added) – Black Beans, Garbanzo Beans, Kidney Beans, Lentil, Lima Beans, Navy Beans, Peas, Pinto Beans, Soybeans

Popcorn Kernels

Rice Cakes

Corn Thins

Salad Dressing (You may want to make your own dairy free, no oil salad dressings for optimal health)

Vinegars

Nut Butters – Peanut Butter, Almond Butter, Soy Butter, Sunflower Seed Butter, Cashew Butter

Baking Powder

Arrowroot Powder

Herbs and Spices – Basil, Bay Leaves, Pepper, Cayenne Pepper, Chili Powder, Cilantro, Dill, Crushed Red Pepper, Garlic Powder, Ground Cinnamon, Ground Cumin, Ground Ginger, Italian Seasoning, Marjoram, Nutmeg, Onion Powder, Oregano, Paprika, Parsley, Sage, Salt, Turmeric

A Few Quick Notes

When you are stocking your food feel free to experiment with what you eat and try new things. Over time you will increase your tastes and find new foods that you enjoy. You can keep them on the grocery list if you like it, or remove it if you find you don't like a certain food.

Use the products that are high in fat and sodium sparingly. Use less dressing and condiments in your food as they can really add on the calories! Chances are you don't really require as much as you've been putting on your food or that you can find an alternative by using herbs, spices, or lemon juice. Give it a try.

It's easiest to plan out what you should buy while figuring out what you'll be eating day by day. When you're making a grocery list you can also plan out the meals that you'll eat that week so that you know exactly what you need to restock up on at the grocery store. Eventually you'll know exactly what you need to prepare the foods that you enjoy eating, but since you're first starting this diet it can be a little difficult. It will be easier to find all of the nutritious foods that you enjoy with time.

Conclusion

What's in the food that you eat daily? Is it filled with the nutrients that help fight and reduce the risk of disease, or is it the reason for all of your health problems? Hopefully now that you have read Designed 2 Eat: The Overall Guide To Health For Life you understand just how important eating really is for your body.

Your lifestyle is in your hands. No one can change the foods that you eat, the exercise routine you keep, or the health problems you face but you. If you're looking to get to the route of your problems, hopefully you've found the solution right here in this book.

Starting a new diet, changing your routine, and adopting a new lifestyle isn't easy. It takes a lot of dedication and hard work. Just know that if you ever slip up, you can easily return to your diet. Every small change adds up, and I totally believe that you can make the necessary changes to live a happier, healthier life.

This book is about happiness, longevity, and understanding how to live the best life you can. I believe that this all begins with the foods that are on your plate.

You know yourself better than anyone else. Do whatever it takes to see success with your new lifestyle. If you're one of those people who has to take a dive in the deep in, then do it! Get rid of all the toxic and unhealthy foods that are sitting in your pantry and start over. It'll be a great experience of learning about new foods, trying new recipes, and taking control of your health.

If you're someone who needs gradual change over time, relax, and plan out how you'd like to start your new lifestyle. There's no right or wrong way to do it except if you don't end up actually committing to the change.

You can take as much time as you need and just start by eating one healthy meal a day. There's no time limit for you to complete this in and I want you to set yourself up for a successful lifelong change.

Begin by planning out the plant-based meals you'd enjoy eating for just one meal and the next time you're shopping purchase the food you want to make and notice how easy it is. Being healthy really is just about making a conscious decision and following through with it. You're going to eat food every day for the rest of your life anyway, so why not have it be as nutritious as it can be?

Within a short time you'll notice all of the health benefits that come from eating a wide range of nutritious foods that you've never experienced with a animal-based high fat diet. Within a matter of weeks you will have lost weight, reduced the chance of developing cancer and cardiovascular disease, lowered your bad cholesterol levels, and decreased your blood sugar levels by successfully eating food that gives you a steady flow of energy throughout the day.

There's nothing better than when you realize a diet is working for you. I promise it will feel so good that you'll never want to go back to eating meat, dairy products, or high fat foods again.

When you get to that point make sure that you share your experiences with others and let them know how they can take control of their health too.

I wish you the best on your journey, and am excited for you to be the healthiest individual you can be. If you need any help throughout your journey, I have added a list of resources that helped contribute to this book, and can clear up any questions about a whole foods plant-

based diet that you might
have.

Resources

Books
The Forks Over Knives Plan – A 4-Week Meal-By-Meal Makeover by Alona Pulde, MD and Matthew Lederman, MD
The China Study by Thomas Campbell and T. Colin Campbell
Whole: Rethinking the Science of Nutrition by T. Colin Campbell and Howard Jacobson
The Complete Idiot's Guide To Plant-Based Nutrition by Julieanna Hever
Unprocessed: How To Achieve Vibrant Health And Your Ideal Weight by Chef AJ and Glen Merzer
The Pleasure Trap: Mastering the Hidden Force that Undermines Health and Happiness by Douglas J. Lisle and Alan Goldhamer
Nutrition for Life: The No-Fad, No-Nonsense Approach To Eating Well And Reaching Your Ideal Weight by Dr. Darwin Deen and Lisa Hark
The Earth Diet by Liana Werner-Gray
Videos
Forks Over Knives
Forks Over Knives Extended Interviews
Forks Over Knives Presents: The Engine 2 Kitchen Rescue
The Veg Edge

Websites
Forks Over Knives, http://www.forksoverknives.com/
Care2 Healthy Living, http://www.care2.com/greenliving/
Everyday Health, http:// www.everydayhealth.com/
Authority Nutrition, http://authoritynutrition.com/
BBC Good Food, http://www.bbcgoodfood.com/e
WebMD, http://www.webmd.com/